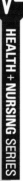

HEALTH + NURSING SERIES

Clinical Dosage Calculations

4TH EDITION

VANESSA BROTTO

KATE RAFFERTY

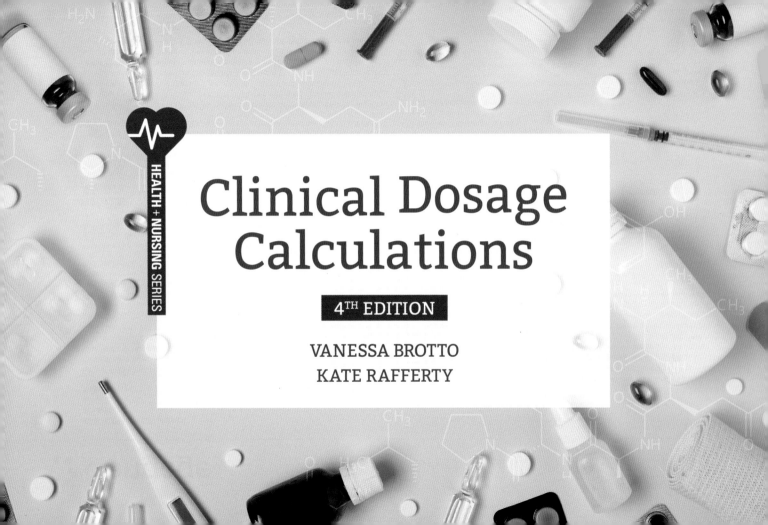

HEALTH + NURSING SERIES

Clinical Dosage Calculations

4TH EDITION

VANESSA BROTTO

KATE RAFFERTY

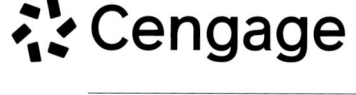

Clinical Dosage Calculations
4th Edition
Vanessa Brotto
Kate Rafferty

Senior Product manager: Michelle Aarons
Content developer: Kylie Scott
Assistant Content project manager: Garima Singh
Text designer: Cengage Creative Studio
Cover designer: Nikita Bansal
Project designer: Nikita Bansal
Editor: Julie Wicks
Proofreader: Anne Mulvaney
Permissions/Photo researcher: Lumina Datamatics
Cover: Adobe/LIGHTFIELD STUDIOS
Typeset by KGL

Any URLs contained in this publication were checked for currency during the production process. Note, however, that the publisher cannot vouch for the ongoing currency of URLs.

Third edition published in 2020

Notice to the Reader
Publisher does not warrant or guarantee any of the products described herein or perform any independent analysis in connection with any of the product information contained herein. Publisher does not assume, and expressly disclaims, any obligation to obtain and include information other than that provided to it by the manufacturer. The reader is expressly warned to consider and adopt all safety precautions that might be indicated by the activities described herein and to avoid all potential hazards. By following the instructions contained herein, the reader willingly assumes all risks in connection with such instructions. The publisher makes no representations or warranties of any kind, including but not limited to, the warranties of fitness for particular purpose or merchantability, nor are any such representations implied with respect to the material set forth herein, and the publisher takes no responsibility with respect to such material. The publisher shall not be liable for any special, consequential, or exemplary damages resulting, in whole or part, from the readers' use of, or reliance upon, this material.

For product information and technology assistance,
in Australia call **1300 790 853**;
in New Zealand call **0800 449 725**

For permission to use material from this text or product, please email
aust.permissions@cengage.com

National Library of Australia Cataloguing-in-Publication Data
ISBN: 9780170465229
A catalogue record for this book is available from the National Library of Australia

Cengage Learning Australia
Level 7, 80 Dorcas Street
South Melbourne, Victoria Australia 3205

For learning solutions, visit **cengage.com.au**

Printed in China by 1010 Printing International Limited.
1 2 3 4 5 6 7 27 26 25 24

PHOTOCOPYING OF BOOKS IS RESTRICTED UNDER LAW

BRIEF CONTENTS

CONTENTS

Part 2 – Skills deepening   144

Part 3 – Skills practice   240

ABOUT THE BOOK

Dosage calculations have often been a source of stress for students and practising health professionals. They are a vital part of clinical practice and can have tragic consequences if performed incorrectly (i.e. if clients inadvertently receive too much or too little of their medications). The response to the previous editions of this book has been overwhelming, with so many students finding dosage calculations much easier when they have some choice over how they approach them.

In formal classes or in other texts, students are often not given a choice as to the method they use when learning how to perform dosage calculations. As a result, many health professionals are taught the 'formula method' only, and they may struggle to remember all the necessary formulae, and how and when to use them. *Clinical Dosage Calculations* allows for variety in the calculations and covers both the formula method and the proportions method (using basic mathematics and ratio principles to solve dosage calculations). This targets those students who struggle with formulae and who might wish to try a different approach.

We have tried to ground this text in the realities of clinical practice by using real-life cases, examples and medicine labels, where possible. Important national concepts and initiatives such as 'risk management' and 'quality use of medicines' are introduced in terms of their application to performing dosage calculations. This allows students to increase their familiarity with the whole process of medicine administration and see the relevance of what they are learning. However, it is beyond the scope of this text to act as a pharmacology resource or medicine administration guide: other relevant texts are needed for these purposes. This book only offers a basic overview of some of these important areas where appropriate.

Clinical Dosage Calculations introduces some unique approaches to the medication chart for the health professional. The '10 steps for safe use of a medication chart' ensures an overall systematic process for calculating doses and establishing which medicines are due/available to administer to a client. The text also incorporates specialist area chapters (midwifery, critical care and paediatrics, with a combined chapter on aged care, mental health and oncology), which allow the reader to practise calculations commonly found in these areas, giving a clinical basis for their learning.

This text may be read from 'front to back' or the reader may choose to skip the general mathematics section and start from the general calculations. It would be advisable for readers to read through the general chapters first before the specialist ones, but this is not strictly required. Each chapter explains the main concepts and shows worked examples. The reader can then engage in the activities of each chapter as an introduction to the concept before moving onto the final chapter, where they can test their knowledge overall. The worked solutions to the activities are available on the companion website and the quick answers may now be found at the back of the book.

We hope you enjoy reading and using *Clinical Dosage Calculations* in your learning, and that the different approaches help with performing calculations.

ABOUT THE AUTHORS

Vanessa Brotto, RN, BN, BAppSci(HP), GDipAdvNurs(CritCare), GCertHigherEd, MClinNurs, was a university academic, for 17 years, having led teaching teams in the Bachelor of Nursing degree, the Postgraduate Diploma of Critical Care and the Master of Nursing Practice (Nurse Practitioner) degrees. She has worked as a clinical nurse specialist in intensive care and post-anaesthetic care units at a major metropolitan hospital in Melbourne, as well as in clinical education for many years. Vanessa has a passion for using diverse teaching methods and making the classroom a fun and engaging learning space. Vanessa won a university teaching award for her approach to teaching large classes and has received a number of university commendations for excellence in teaching.

Vanessa is currently serving her third term as a core member of the Scheduled Medicines Expert Committee for the Australian Health Practitioner Regulation Agency (AHPRA), advising national boards on their use of scheduled medicines both generally and when developing submissions for endorsements by the Australian Health Workforce Ministerial Council.

Kate Rafferty, RN, DipAppSci(Nurs), GCertPaed(CritCare), GCertNursAcuteCare(Periop Pract), Cert IV TAA, is currently the Business Development Manager for RPS Australia, working as the Melbourne-based clinic nurse and a perioperative nurse in Southwest Healthcare. Kate also has experience lecturing at Deakin University, teaching in the Certificate IV of Nursing and coordinating several traineeships in health-affiliated areas across Victoria with South West TAFE. She has worked as a registered nurse in cardiac intensive care in the Royal Alexandra Hospital for Children in Sydney and as a perioperative nurse at St Vincent's and St Vincent's Private Hospitals in Melbourne. She has experience in a coordinator's role at St John of God in Warrnambool, as a unit manager in aged care and as a Director of Nursing in rural south-west Victoria. Kate has a strong interest in making health education vibrant and memorable.

ACKNOWLEDGEMENTS

The fourth edition of this book would not have been possible without the support of our great team at Cengage Learning and our family and colleagues. The team at Cengage have been a pleasure to work with – a special thank you to Michelle Aarons (content manager), Kylie Scott (content developer) and Julie Wicks (copyeditor), who have been a brilliant team to work with. Thanks must also go to our external reviewers who gave valuable feedback and advice on each of the chapters in order to improve the relevance of the text in Australia and New Zealand.

From Vanessa: I could not have done this without the support of my amazing family and friends. I dedicate this work to my two daughters Aniela and Amalie, who have been a constant source of laughter and support.

From Kate: To my wonderful family and friends – thank you. Your ongoing support, encouragement and understanding continue to give me the energy to meet deadlines.

Vanessa Brotto and Kate Rafferty

Cengage Learning would like to thank Deborah Pidd (RN, RM, MMID, PhD candidate, Latrobe University) for her contribution to the midwifery chapter, and Elise Worland (RN, Cert IV Training & Assessment, Dip Vocational Education & Training) for her contribution to the chapter on specialist areas of aged care, mental health and oncology. The authors and Cengage would also like to thank the following reviewers for their incisive and helpful feedback:

- Lin Zhao, RMIT
- Tanya Langtree, James Cook University
- Charlotte George, Employease
- Sonja Dawson, Avondale College
- Joclyn Neal, Australian Catholic University
- Aaron Grogan, University of Queensland
- Bronwyn Garroch, University of Queensland
- Rita Eramo, Victoria University
- Srinivas Nammi, Western Sydney University

Guide to the text

As you read this text you will find a number of features in every chapter to enhance your study of clinical dosage calculations.

FEATURES WITHIN CHAPTERS

Find the information to correctly calculate and administer drug doses with examples using **real medication charts and medication labels**.

Date	Warfarin		Marevan/Coumadin select brand		INR Result											
Route	Prescriber to enter individual doses		Target INR Range		**Dose**	mg	mg	mg	mg	mg	mg	mg	mg	mg	mg
Indication			Pharmacy		Prescriber										
		Print your name		Contact	*1600* Initial 1										
					Initial 2										

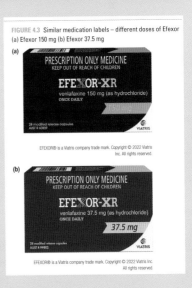

FIGURE 4.3 Similar medication labels – different doses of Efexor (a) Efexor 150 mg (b) Efexor 37.5 mg

Worked examples demonstrate how to work out the key calculations that you will need to accurately administer medications.

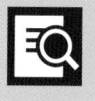 **Clinical case study icons** identify where real-life scenarios are used throughout the worked examples and activities.

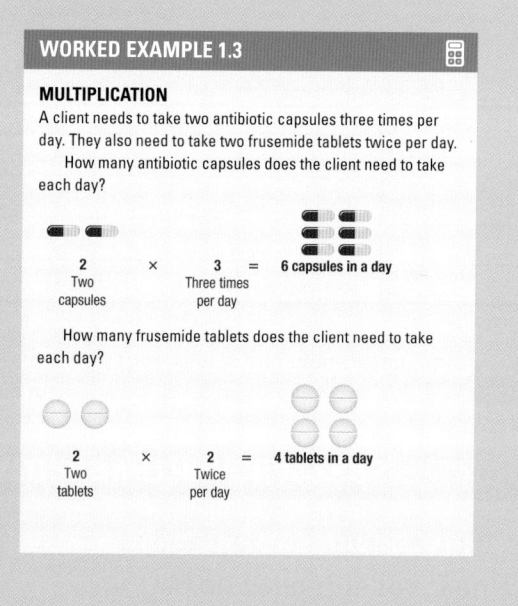

WORKED EXAMPLE 1.3

MULTIPLICATION

A client needs to take two antibiotic capsules three times per day. They also need to take two frusemide tablets twice per day.

How many antibiotic capsules does the client need to take each day?

| **2**
Two
capsules | × | **3**
Three times
per day | = | **6 capsules in a day** |

How many frusemide tablets does the client need to take each day?

| **2**
Two
tablets | × | **2**
Twice
per day | = | **4 tablets in a day** |

Reinforce your knowledge of safety tips and procedures with the **Safety** boxes.

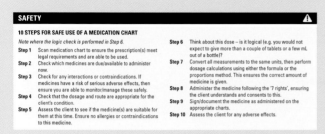

Formula boxes highlight important mathematical concepts.

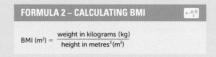

Test your understanding of concepts and practise calculations with the **activities**.

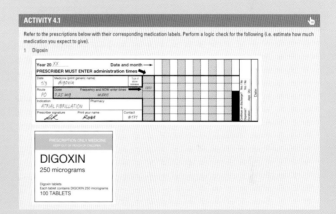

Refer to the **useful formulae** printed on the inside covers to help with your revision.

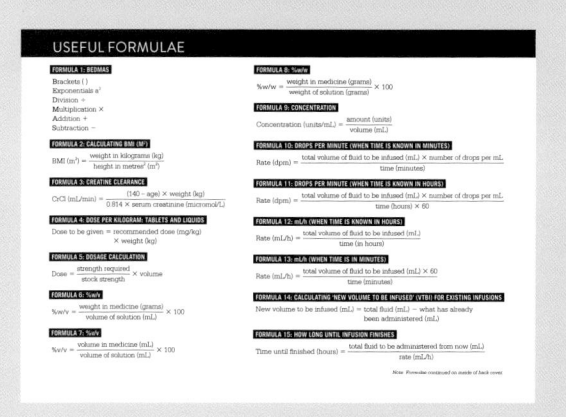

END OF BOOK FEATURES

At the end of the book you will find:

- **Practice questions** to test your skills
- Brief **answers** to selected questions from the text
- An **index** to help you locate key terms and concepts.

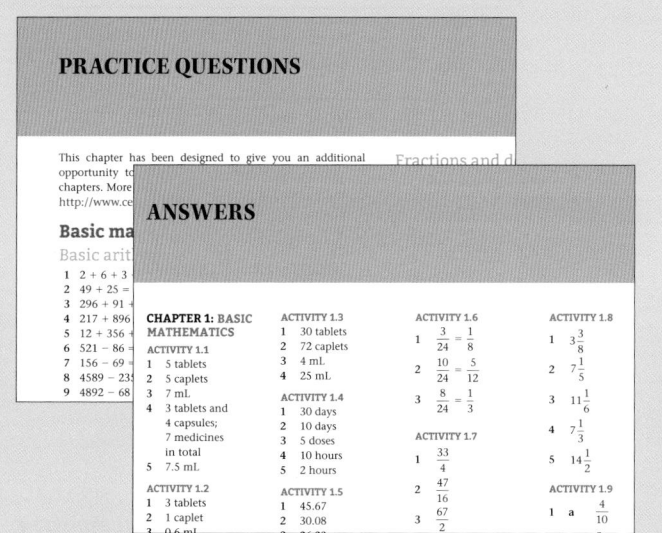

Guide to the online resources

FOR THE INSTRUCTOR

Cengage is pleased to provide you with a selection of resources that will help you prepare your lectures and assessments when you choose this textbook for your course. Log in or request an account to access instructor resources at **au.cengage.com/instructor/account** for Australia or **nz.cengage.com/instructor/account** for New Zealand.

MINDTAP

Premium online teaching and learning tools are available on the *MindTap* platform - the personalised eLearning solution.

MindTap is a flexible and easy-to-use platform that helps build student confidence and gives you a clear picture of their progress. We partner with you to ease the transition to digital – we're with you every step of the way.

MindTap for Clinical Dosage Calculations is full of innovative resources to support critical thinking, and help your students move from memorisation to mastery! Includes:

* *Clinical Dosage Calculations* eBook

* revision quizzes for skills practice

* real medication charts and real medication labels

* videos that step you through key concepts

MindTap is a premium purchasable eLearning tool. Contact your Cengage learning consultant to find out how MindTap can transform your course.

SOLUTIONS MANUAL

The solutions manual includes a full set of worked solutions for each chapter activity.

POWERPOINT PRESENTATIONS

Use the chapter-by-chapter PowerPoint presentations to enhance your lecture presentations and to reinforce the key principles of your subject, or for student handouts.

COGNERO TEST BANK

A bank of questions has been developed in conjunction with the text for creating quizzes, tests and exams for your students. Create multiple test versions in an instant and deliver tests from your LMS, your classroom, or wherever you want using Cognero. Cognero test generator is a flexible online system that allows you to import, edit and manipulate content from the text's test bank or elsewhere, including your own favourite test questions.

ARTWORK FROM THE TEXT

Add the digital files of graphs, pictures and flowcharts into your course management system, use them in student handouts or copy them into lecture presentations.

MINDTAP

MindTap is the next-level online learning tool that helps you get better grades!

MindTap gives you the resources you need to study – all in one place and available when you need them. In the *MindTap Reader*, you can make notes, highlight text and even find a definition directly from the page.

If your instructor has chosen *MindTap* for your subject this semester, log in to *MindTap* to:

- Get better grades
- Save time and get organised
- Connect with your instructor and peers
- Study when and where you want, online and mobile
- Complete assessment tasks as set by your instructor.
- When your instructor creates a course using *MindTap*, they will let you know your course key so you can access the content. Please purchase *MindTap* only when directed by your instructor. Course length is set by your instructor.

PART 1

FUNDAMENTAL SKILLS

1

CHAPTER 1 — BASIC MATHEMATICS

Introduction

Basic mathematics is a vital skill for health professionals who are administering medicines to clients. In order to learn and master dosage calculations, the clinician must be able to apply mathematical principles concerning arithmetic, fractions, ratios and percentages.

Later chapters in this text discuss the approaches to solving dosage calculations using either a formula or a proportions method. Both of these require a good understanding and ability to apply mathematical principles.

This chapter introduces the relevant mathematics to support both the proportions and the formulae methods for calculation that will be introduced in Chapter 5.

Basic arithmetic

'Basic arithmetic' is a term used to describe the general mathematics used by most people in society on a daily basis. It incorporates addition, subtraction, multiplication and division of whole numbers.

Addition (+)

Addition is the sum or combining of numbers together. It uses the addition symbol '+' and can be seen in **Figure 1.1** showing that one tablet plus two tablets adds up to three tablets. Words that indicate addition include 'add', 'plus', 'combine' and 'sum'. Addition is the opposite of subtraction.

FIGURE 1.1 Addition: 1 tablet + 2 tablets = 3 tablets

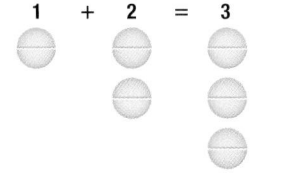

WORKED EXAMPLE 1.1

ADDITION

A client asks you how many medicines they need to swallow to take all their morning medicines. They have the following medicines to take:

- 500 mg paracetamol (2 capsules)
- 40 mg frusemide (1 tablet)
- 62.5 microg digoxin (2 tablets)
- 100 mg aspirin (1 tablet)
- 500 mg amoxycillin (1 capsule)

How many tablets does the client need to take?

First we look at which medicines are in tablet form from the list above:

frusemide	(1 tablet)		1
digoxin	(2 tablets)		+2
aspirin	(1 tablet)		+1
			4 tablets in total

How many capsules does the client need to take?

First we look at which medicines are in capsule form from the list above:

amoxycillin	(1 capsule)		1
paracetamol	(2 capsules)		+2
			3 capsules in total

How many medicines in total does the client need to take (i.e. total including all tablets and capsules)?

Now we look at ALL the tablets and capsules together and add them all up:

frusemide	(1 tablet)		1
digoxin	(2 tablets)		+2
aspirin	(1 tablet)		+1
amoxycillin	(1 capsule)		+1
paracetamol	(2 capsules)		+2
			7 in total

ACTIVITY 1.1

Add up the following:

1   How many tablets are there?

2   How many caplets are there?

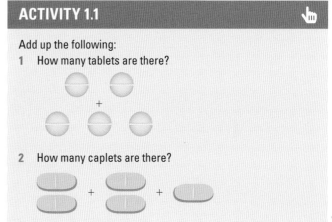

>>

>>

3 How many millilitres (mL) of saline are there in total in these syringes?

4 How many tablets are there? How many capsules are there? How many in total?

5 How many mL of liquid are there in total?

Subtraction (−)

Subtraction is the removal or 'taking away' of one number from another. It uses the symbol '−' and can be seen in Figure 1.2 showing that if there were four tablets and three were subtracted, then there would only be one tablet left. In dosage calculations, it is important to ensure that the smaller number is subtracted from the bigger number. Words that indicate subtraction include 'subtract', 'minus', 'take away' and 'remove'. Subtraction is the opposite of addition.

FIGURE 1.2 Subtraction: 4 tablets − 3 tablets = 1 tablet

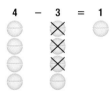

WORKED EXAMPLE 1.2

SUBTRACTION

A nurse needs to administer 'Coloxyl and Senna' tablets to three clients. The nurse then needs to calculate how many tablets will be left in the bottle to see if more need to be ordered from the pharmacy department. There are 25 tablets in the bottle at the start of the day.

The first client is ordered one 'Coloxyl and Senna' tablet. How many tablets will be left in the bottle?

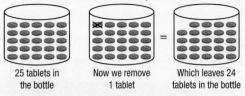

First we look at what we have in total (i.e. 25 tablets in this bottle).

25 tablets in the bottle / Now we remove 1 tablet / Which leaves 24 tablets in the bottle

How many tablets are left in the bottle if the second client requires two tablets?

After the first client took 1 tablet, we only have 24 tablets left in this bottle.

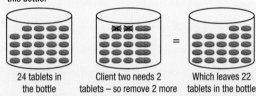

24 tablets in the bottle / Client two needs 2 tablets – so remove 2 more / Which leaves 22 tablets in the bottle

How many tablets are left in the bottle if the third client requires four tablets?

After the first client took 1 tablet and then the second client took 2 tablets, we only have 22 tablets left in this bottle.

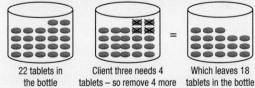

22 tablets in the bottle / Client three needs 4 tablets – so remove 4 more / Which leaves 18 tablets in the bottle

ACTIVITY 1.2

Calculate the following:

1 How many tablets are there if two are removed?

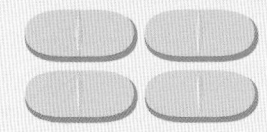

2 How many caplets are there if three are subtracted?

3 How many millilitres of saline is left in this syringe if 1.4 mL is subtracted?

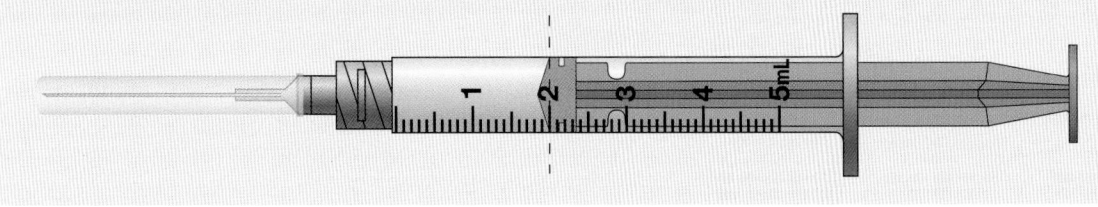

>>

4 How many capsules are left if you 'take away' five of them?

5 How many mL of paracetamol liquid is left in a 200 mL bottle if you remove 5.5 mL?

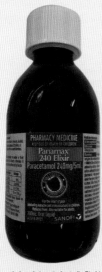

© Sanofi-Aventis Australia Pty Ltd

Multiplication (×)

In basic terms, multiplication is a short-cut way to add up numbers. It is the way we calculate the total combination of a group of numbers. It uses the symbol '×' and can be seen in Figure 1.3 showing that if there were two medicine cups that each contained three tablets, then we could multiply three by two to find we have a total of six tablets. Words that indicate multiplication include 'multiply', 'times' and 'by' (i.e. two by three equals six). Multiplication is the opposite of division.

FIGURE 1.3 Multiplication: 3 tablets × 2 lots = 6 tablets or 3 × 2 = 6 tablets

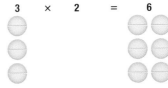

3   ×   2   =   6

i.e. This is the first lot of 3 | Multiplied by 2 | Together they make a total of 6

Multiplying by 1, 10, 100, 1000

Multiplying a number by 1 does not change anything as the number remains the same; however, when you multiply a number by 10 you need to add a zero after the number. For example:

$6 \times 1 = 6$ (i.e. it does not change)

$6 \times 10 = 60$ (i.e. the 6 remains but we add a zero, making the answer 60)

$6 \times 100 = 600$ (i.e. we add two zeros, as this is the number of zeros found in 100)

$6 \times 1000 = 6000$ (i.e. we add three zeros, as this is the number of zeros found in 1000)

WORKED EXAMPLE 1.3

MULTIPLICATION

A client needs to take two antibiotic capsules three times per day. They also need to take two frusemide tablets twice per day.

How many antibiotic capsules does the client need to take each day?

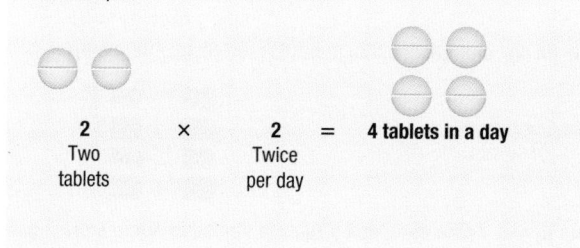

| **2**
Two
capsules | × | **3**
Three times
per day | = | **6 capsules in a day** |

How many frusemide tablets does the client need to take each day?

| **2**
Two
tablets | × | **2**
Twice
per day | = | **4 tablets in a day** |

How many frusemide tablets in total does the client need if they go away on holiday for six days?

From the previous question, we know the client needs $2 \times 2 = 4$ frusemide tablets each day.

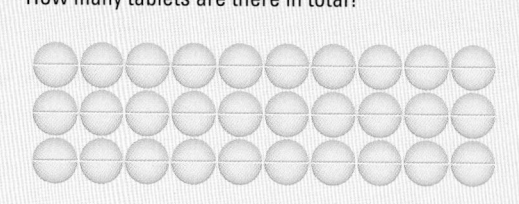

Day 1
Day 2
Day 3
Day 4
Day 5
Day 6

| **4**
Four tablets
each day | × | **6**
By six
days | = | **24 tablets needed in total** |

ACTIVITY 1.3

Multiply the following:

1   How many tablets are there in total?

>>

2 How many Efexor capsules are there if you have three packets?

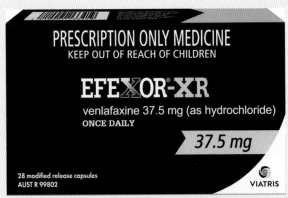

3 How many millilitres (mL) of saline are there in total in both of these syringes?

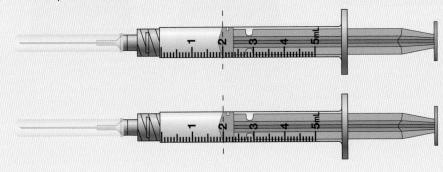

>>

4 How many mL of liquid are there altogether?

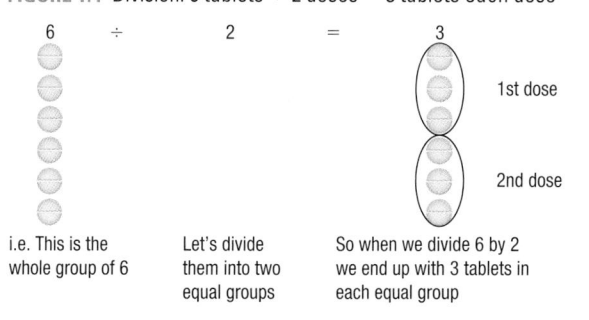

FIGURE 1.4 Division: 6 tablets ÷ 2 doses = 3 tablets each dose

6   ÷   2   =   3

1st dose

2nd dose

i.e. This is the whole group of 6

Let's divide them into two equal groups

So when we divide 6 by 2 we end up with 3 tablets in each equal group

Division (÷)

Division is a way to work out how many times something is contained in a group. It uses the symbol '÷' and can be seen in Figure 1.4 showing that if there were six tablets in a cup, then we could divide those up into two medicine cups containing three tablets each. Words that indicate division include 'divide', 'go into' and 'separate'. Division is the opposite of multiplication.

WORKED EXAMPLE 1.4

DIVISION

A client needs to reduce the number of prednisolone tablets they take each day as part of their treatment. On Monday they need to take four tablets and they need to reduce this by half each day.

How many tablets does the client need to take on Tuesday?

Monday: four tablets

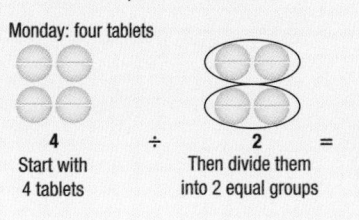

4   ÷   2   =   **2 tablets on Tuesday**
Start with   Then divide them   Which gives 2 groups of
4 tablets   into 2 equal groups   TWO tablets so this means
                                                      the answer to 4 ÷ 2 = 2

>>

How many tablets does the client need to take on Wednesday?

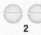

2	÷	2	=	1 tablet on Wednesday
Start with		Then divide them		Which gives 2 groups of ONE
2 tablets		into 2 equal groups		tablet so this means the answer
				to 2 ÷ 2 = 1

Dividing by 1, 10, 100, 1000

Dividing a number by 1 does not change anything as the number remains the same; however, when you divide a number by 10 you need to remove a zero after the number. For example:

$6000 \div 1 = 6000$ (i.e. it does not change)

$6000 \div 10 = 600$ (i.e. we remove one zero, as this is the number of zeros in 10)

$6000 \div 100 = 60$ (i.e. we remove two zeros, as this is the number of zeros found in 100)

$6000 \div 1000 = 6$ (i.e. we remove three zeros, as this is the number of zeros found in 1000)

ACTIVITY 1.4

Divide the following:

1 A client requires two puffs of their fluticasone inhaler each day. The inhaler contains 60 doses. How many days will this inhaler last?

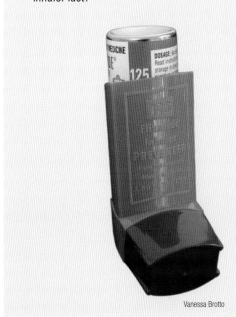

Vanessa Brotto

\>\>

>>

2 A client is ordered 20 mL of lactulose syrup once a day. How many days will the 200 mL bottle last?

3 A vial of a medicine is made up to a total of 10 mL. A client requires 2 mL doses. How many doses are in the vial for this single client?

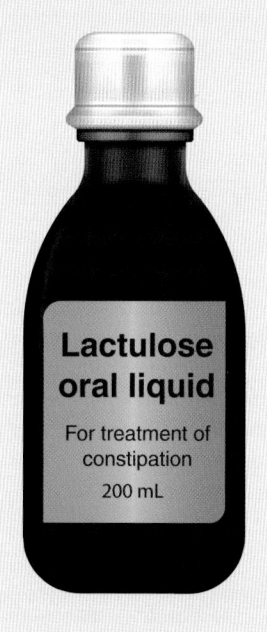

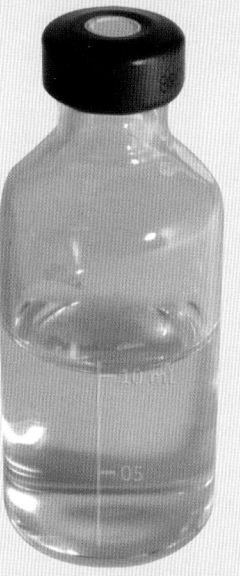

Robert Byron/Dreamstime LLC

4   The nurse checks to see how much intravenous fluid is left in a client's burette. It is running at 10 mL per hour. How many hours will it take for this fluid to be finished?

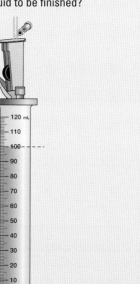

5   The nurse checks to see how much intravenous fluid is left in a client's burette. It is running at 50 mL per hour. How many hours will it take for this fluid to be finished?

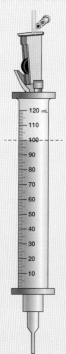

Order of operations (BEDMAS)

When a mathematical problem requires more than one simple operation at a time, it is important to do the steps in the correct order so as to obtain the correct answer. There are a number of acronyms to help remember these steps but, basically, they show the same sequence: you perform the calculations in brackets first, then you do any exponentials, then division, followed by multiplication, and then lastly the addition and subtraction.

FORMULA 1 – BEDMAS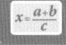

Brackets ( )
Exponentials a^2
Division ÷
Multiplication ×
Addition +
Subtraction −

FORMULA 2 – CALCULATING BMI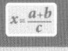

$$BMI \ (m^2) = \frac{\text{weight in kilograms (kg)}}{\text{height in metres}^2 \ (m^2)}$$

WORKED EXAMPLE 1.5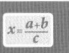

ORDER OF OPERATIONS (BEDMAS)

A client weighs 91 kg and is 1.8 m tall. The health professional needs to calculate their body mass index (BMI).

Using Formula 2, how do we calculate this using the correct sequence or order of operations?

Brackets	There are none to calculate here
Exponentials	Calculate the height in metres^2 first

$$1.8 \ m \times 1.8 \ m = 3.24 \ m^2$$

Division	Then do the division component

$$BMI \ (m^2) = \frac{91 \ kg}{3.24 \ m^2} \quad \text{or } 91 \div 3.24 = 28.09$$

Multiplication	There are none to calculate here
Addition	There are none to calculate here
Subtraction	There are none to calculate here

FORMULA 3 – CREATININE CLEARANCE

$$CrCl \ (mL/min) = \frac{(140 - age) \times \text{weight (kg)}}{0.814 \times \text{serum creatinine (micromol / L)}}$$

Calculate the following:

1 Calculate the body mass index (BMI) of Mr Basil Savoy (weight = 132 kg, height = 1.7 m) using this formula:

$$\text{BMI (m}^2) = \frac{\text{weight in kilograms}}{\text{height in metres}^2}$$

2 Calculate the body mass index (BMI) of Mrs Patricia Norman (weight = 77 kg, height = 1.6 m) using this formula:

$$\text{BMI (m}^2) = \frac{\text{weight in kilograms}}{\text{height in metres}^2}$$

3 Calculate the body mass index (BMI) of Mr Jonathon Vincents (weight = 85 kg, height = 1.8 m) using this formula:

$$\text{BMI (m}^2) = \frac{\text{weight in kilograms}}{\text{height in metres}^2}$$

4 Calculate the creatinine clearance (CrCl) of Mr Isidoro Scarbossa, aged 80 years. His serum creatinine is 465 micromol/L and his ideal body weight is 57 kg. You will need to use Formula 3, which is from *Therapeutic Guidelines: Antibiotic* for males.

Fractions and decimals

Fractions

What are fractions?

A fraction is a number that is expressed in two parts. The top part of the number is the amount of parts that are present, and the bottom number tells you how many parts there are in the whole. The top number is called the 'numerator' and the bottom number is called the 'denominator' (see Figure 1.5).

Proper fractions

A proper fraction is a fraction that has a numerator smaller than the denominator (example $\frac{5}{12}$ or $\frac{1}{2}$ or $\frac{3}{4}$).

FIGURE 1.5 One-quarter of a tablet

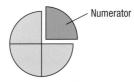

Numerator

■ One-quarter $(\frac{1}{4})$
■ Three-quarters $(\frac{3}{4})$

In this diagram, the numerator for the dark green section is 1 and the denominator is 4.

WORKED EXAMPLE 1.6

Another example using everyday terms is to look at a block of chocolate with 24 squares.

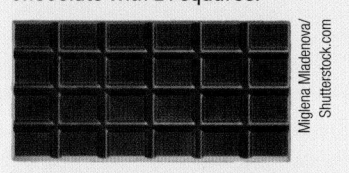

Miglena Mladenova/Shutterstock.com

If we were to eat 5 squares of chocolate, expressed as a fraction, the numerator is 5, as part of a whole 24 (denominator).

This would be expressed as $\frac{5}{24}$

ACTIVITY 1.6

Using the same example (Worked example 1.6), express the following as a fraction:

1   Express 3 squares of chocolate as a fraction of the whole block.
2   Express 10 squares of chocolate as a fraction of the whole block.
3   Express 8 squares of chocolate as a fraction of the whole block.

Mixed fractions or mixed numbers

A mixed fraction is also known as a 'mixed number'. It is a combination of a whole number and a proper fraction. This concept is no more complicated than considering buying 2 pizzas and eating 1 full pizza and $\frac{1}{4}$ of another = $1\frac{1}{4}$.

Examples of mixed fractions are $3\frac{3}{8}$, $8\frac{1}{4}$, $2\frac{15}{16}$, $33\frac{1}{2}$.

Improper fractions

An improper fraction is a fraction that has its numerator equal to or larger than the denominator. Examples of improper fractions are $\frac{19}{12}$, $\frac{32}{12}$, $\frac{12}{12}$. Improper fractions, when broken down, have their answer as a mixed fraction. In order to change improper fractions to mixed fractions, we need to divide the denominator into the numerator (see Worked example 1.8).

Converting mixed fractions to improper fractions

There are three steps to converting mixed fractions into improper fractions:

Step 1   Multiply the whole number by the denominator.
Step 2   Add the numerator to this number.
Step 3   Write down the number above the denominator.

WORKED EXAMPLE 1.7

MIXED NUMBERS

Convert the mixed number $3\frac{5}{8}$ to an improper fraction:

Step 1 Multiply the whole number by the denominator

$3 \times 8 = 24$

Step 2 Add the numerator to this number

$24 + 5 = 29$

Step 3 Write down the number above the denominator

$\frac{29}{8}$

ACTIVITY 1.7

Convert the following mixed fractions to improper fractions:

1 $8\frac{1}{4}$ 4 $16\frac{2}{8}$

2 $2\frac{15}{16}$ 5 $8\frac{5}{7}$

3 $33\frac{1}{2}$

Converting improper fractions to mixed fractions

There are three steps to converting improper fractions into mixed fractions.

Step 1 Divide the numerator by the denominator.
Step 2 Write down the whole number answer.
Step 3 Write down any remainder above the denominator.

WORKED EXAMPLE 1.8

IMPROPER FRACTIONS

Convert the following improper fractions into mixed numbers using the following steps:

Step 1 Divide the numerator by the denominator.
Step 2 Write down the whole number answer.
Step 3 Write down any remainder above the denominator.

a $\frac{19}{12} = 1\frac{7}{12}$ When 12 is divided into 19, we get 1 as a whole number and $\frac{7}{12}$ left over.

b $\frac{32}{12} = 2\frac{8}{12}$ When 12 is divided into 32, we get 2 as a whole number and $\frac{8}{12}$ left over.

c $\frac{12}{12} = 1$ When 12 is divided into 12, we get 1 as a whole number.

ACTIVITY 1.8

Convert the following improper fractions to mixed numbers:

1 $\dfrac{27}{8}$ 4 $\dfrac{22}{3}$

2 $\dfrac{36}{5}$ 5 $\dfrac{29}{2}$

3 $\dfrac{67}{6}$

Cancelling equivalent fractions

An equivalent fraction is a fraction that has the same value, regardless of how it is presented. Figure 1.6 shows that if you eat a quarter of a piece of cake, it is the equivalent of eating $\dfrac{2}{8}$ of the second cake. The second cake is merely cut into more pieces.

FIGURE 1.6 Equivalent fractions

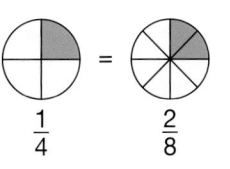

The relationship between the two fractions is that both the numerator and the denominator have been multiplied by 2.

WORKED EXAMPLE 1.9

EQUIVALENT FRACTIONS

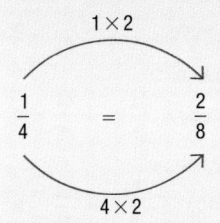

When cancelling equivalent fractions that include whole numbers, the format and the rules remain the same.

Consider the two diagrams that involve two tablets: one tablet remains whole and the other tablet has been split into pieces.

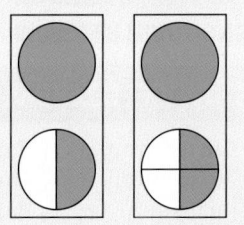

One and one-half $\left(1\dfrac{1}{2}\right)$ tablets on the left is the same as one and two-quarter $\left(1\dfrac{2}{4}\right)$ tablets on the right.

>>

On the left, there is one whole green tablet and one tablet split into two pieces (one green piece and one yellow piece).

On the right, there is one whole green tablet and one tablet split into four pieces (two green pieces and two yellow pieces).

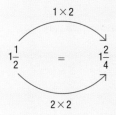

In this example, $1\frac{1}{2}$ is equivalent to $1\frac{2}{4}$. You can make equivalent fractions by multiplying (or dividing) both the numerator and the denominator by the same number. In this case, the numerator and the denominator are both multiplied by 2.

From here, it is an easy step to change equivalent fractions by omitting the diagram step. If it helps, you can still use the arrows until you are comfortable with this presentation.

1 a Split each coloured piece into two.

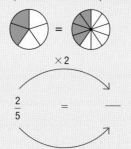

b Split each coloured piece into three.

>>

c   Split each coloured piece into two.

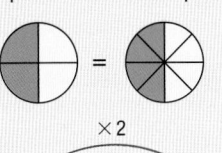

$$\frac{2}{4} = \underline{}$$

d   Split each piece into three.

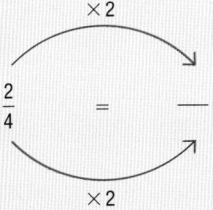

$$\frac{3}{4} = \underline{}$$

e   Split each piece into two.

$$\frac{5}{8} = \underline{}$$

f   Split each piece into three.

$$\frac{5}{9} = \underline{}$$

2   Show the equivalent fraction for the fractions below:

a $\dfrac{1}{2} = \dfrac{}{12}$

b $\dfrac{1}{4} = \dfrac{}{12}$

c $\dfrac{1}{5} = \dfrac{}{60}$

d $\dfrac{7}{8} = \dfrac{}{72}$

e $\dfrac{4}{8} = \dfrac{}{64}$

f $\dfrac{2}{6} = \dfrac{12}{}$

g $\dfrac{2}{5} = \dfrac{10}{}$

The skill of using and working out equivalent fractions is used in the addition, subtraction and comparison of fractions.

How to reduce fractions to their lowest or simplest form

Simplifying fractions to their lowest or simplest form is another important skill. When you simplify or reduce a fraction, you don't change the actual value of the fraction; instead, you are writing it in its smallest form. When writing fractions in their simplest forms, you are required to find the greatest common factor. This is the largest number that evenly divides into both the numerator and the denominator. As mentioned above, the numerator is the top number in a fraction and the denominator is the bottom number. The fraction is simplified when the numerator and the denominator of the fraction share no common factors other than one. This is called a prime number.

An easy example of this follows in Worked example 1.10.

$$\frac{1}{4} + \frac{1}{4} = \frac{2}{4}$$

$$\frac{1}{4} + \frac{1}{4} = \frac{2}{4} = \frac{\overset{1}{\cancel{2}}}{2 \times \cancel{2}_{1}} + \frac{1}{2}$$

In this example, the answer after adding the fractions is $\frac{2}{4}$. To determine the lowest common equivalent fraction, we need to look for the highest number in common as a factor to the numerator and the denominator. When we find these numbers, we can reduce the numerator and denominator to their simplest form.

The number '2' is a common factor to both the numerator and the denominator in this example. This tells us that the fraction is not in its simplest form. The result is a fraction converted to its lowest form $\left(\frac{1}{2}\right)$.

Always keep in mind that whatever you do to the numerator, you must also do to the denominator.

This means that you must always divide both the top and bottom part of a fraction by the same number. This way the overall value of the fraction is not changed. Worked example 1.11 gives a description of how this is done.

$$\frac{18}{24} + \frac{2}{24} = \frac{20}{24}$$

$$\frac{18}{24} + \frac{2}{24} = \frac{20}{\cancel{24}} = \frac{10}{\cancel{12}} = \textcircled{\frac{5}{6}} \longleftarrow \text{Prime number}$$

We add the fraction to get $\frac{20}{24}$ and the factor common to both 20 and 24 is 2. So, 20 divided by 2 is 10 and 24 divided by 2 is 12, giving us $\frac{10}{12}$. We can divide both numbers by a factor of 2 to reduce them to $\frac{5}{6}$. Given that the fraction $\frac{5}{6}$ is not divisible by a common number, then this fraction is in its simplest form.

How to add fractions

There are three steps for adding fractions:

Step 1 Make sure the denominators are the same.
Step 2 Add the numerators.
Step 3 Simplify the fraction.

WORKED EXAMPLE 1.12

EXAMPLE 1

$$\frac{1}{4} + \frac{2}{4}$$

Step 1 Make sure the denominators are the same
Step 2 Add the numerators
Step 3 Simplify the fraction

$$\frac{1}{4} + \frac{2}{4} = \frac{1+2}{4} = \frac{3}{4}$$

EXAMPLE 2

$$\frac{3}{8} + \frac{1}{8} = \frac{3+1}{8} = \frac{4}{8}$$

Step 3 Simplify the fraction
(Remember to reduce the numbers in the fraction to prime numbers where possible)

$$\frac{4}{8} = \frac{2}{4} = \frac{①}{2} \longleftarrow \text{Prime number}$$

EXAMPLE 3

$$\frac{1}{3} + \frac{2}{9}$$

Step 1 Make sure the denominators are the same

$$\frac{1}{3} + \frac{2}{9}$$

Remember multiplying the fraction to make equivalent fractions?

$$\frac{1}{3} + \frac{2}{9} = \frac{1}{3} \quad \xrightarrow{\times 3} \quad \frac{3}{9} + \frac{2}{9}$$
$$\xrightarrow{\times 3}$$

Step 2 Add the numerators

$$\frac{3}{9} + \frac{2}{9} = \frac{5}{9}$$

Step 3 Simplify the fraction

$$\frac{⑤}{9} \longleftarrow \text{Prime number}$$

As you can see, the fraction is already simplified to its smallest form.

ACTIVITY 1.10

Complete the following addition of fraction questions:

1   $\dfrac{3}{4}+\dfrac{1}{4}=$

2   $\dfrac{3}{8}+\dfrac{1}{8}=$

3   $\dfrac{3}{10}+\dfrac{2}{10}=$

4   $\dfrac{2}{7}+\dfrac{1}{21}=$

5   $\dfrac{4}{5}+\dfrac{1}{15}=$

How to subtract fractions

Once again, there are three steps for subtracting fractions:

Step 1   Make sure the denominators are the same.

Step 2   Subtract the numerators.

Step 3   Simplify the fraction.

WORKED EXAMPLE 1.13

EXAMPLE 1

$$\dfrac{3}{4}-\dfrac{1}{4}$$

Step 1   The denominators are the same

Step 2   Subtract the numerators

$$\dfrac{3}{4}-\dfrac{1}{4}=\dfrac{2}{4}$$

Step 3   Simplify the fraction

 $\dfrac{2^{\,1}}{4_{\,2}}=\dfrac{①}{2}$ ←——Prime number

EXAMPLE 2

$$\dfrac{1}{2}-\dfrac{1}{8}$$

Step 1   The denominators are the same

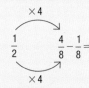

$\overset{\times 4}{\underset{\times 4}{\dfrac{1}{2}}}\quad \dfrac{4}{8}-\dfrac{1}{8}=$

Step 2   Subtract the numerators

$$\dfrac{4}{8}-\dfrac{1}{8}=\dfrac{3}{8}$$

Step 3   Simplify the equation

As 3 is a prime number, this is the simplest the fraction can be.

ACTIVITY 1.11

Complete the following subtraction of fraction questions using the three rules:

1 $\dfrac{5}{9} - \dfrac{1}{6} =$

4 $\dfrac{3}{5} - \dfrac{2}{10} =$

2 $\dfrac{6}{9} - \dfrac{5}{10} =$

5 $\dfrac{2}{5} - \dfrac{1}{9} =$

3 $\dfrac{2}{5} - \dfrac{1}{7} =$

How to multiply fractions

Learning how to multiply fractions is necessary if you decide to use the proportions method of calculating dosages. This method gives you an alternative to using formulae and is covered in this text. There are three steps for multiplying fractions:

Step 1 Multiply the numerators.

Step 2 Multiply the denominators.

Step 3 Simplify the fraction.

WORKED EXAMPLE 1.14

EXAMPLE 1

$$\dfrac{1}{2} \times \dfrac{2}{5}$$

Step 1 Multiply the numerators

Step 2 Multiply the denominators

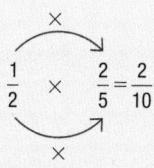

$$\dfrac{1}{2} \times \dfrac{2}{5} = \dfrac{2}{10}$$

Step 3 Simplify the fraction

$$\dfrac{\overset{1}{\cancel{2}}}{\underset{5}{\cancel{10}}} = \dfrac{\textcircled{1}}{5} \longleftarrow \text{Prime number}$$

EXAMPLE 2

$$\dfrac{3}{4} \times \dfrac{1}{3}$$

Step 1 Multiply the numerators

>>

Step 2   Multiply the denominators

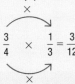

$$\frac{3}{4} \times \frac{1}{3} = \frac{3}{12}$$

Step 3   Simplify the fraction

$$\frac{\cancel{3}^{1}}{\cancel{12}_{4}} = \frac{1}{4}$$

EXAMPLE 3

$$\frac{1}{3} \times \frac{3}{5}$$

Step 1   Multiply the numerators
Step 2   Multiply the denominators

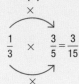

$$\frac{1}{3} \times \frac{3}{5} = \frac{3}{15}$$

Step 3   Simplify the fraction

$$\frac{\cancel{3}^{1}}{\cancel{15}_{5}} = \frac{1}{5}$$

Using the three-step rule, try the following questions:

1   $\dfrac{2}{4} \times \dfrac{1}{8} =$

2   $\dfrac{2}{4} \times \dfrac{3}{4} =$

3   $\dfrac{2}{3} \times \dfrac{4}{6} =$

4   $\dfrac{7}{8} \times \dfrac{6}{8} =$

5   $\dfrac{7}{8} \times \dfrac{7}{9} =$

How to divide fractions

There are three steps for dividing fractions:

Step 1   Take the second fraction (the one that you are dividing by) and turn it upside down (which turns it into a reciprocal). This means that the two numbers when multiplied together will equal one (e.g. $\frac{1}{2} \times \frac{2}{1} = 1$).

Step 2   Multiply the numerators and the denominators (as if you are multiplying fractions).

Step 3   Simplify the fraction.

WORKED EXAMPLE 1.15

To divide $\frac{1}{2}$ by $\frac{1}{6}$ follow the given steps.

Step 1   Turn the divisor fraction into a reciprocal

$$\frac{1}{2} \div \boxed{\frac{1}{6}} \longleftarrow \frac{6}{1}$$

$$\frac{1}{2} \times \frac{6}{1}$$

Step 2   Multiply the numerator and denominator

$$\frac{1}{2} \times \frac{6}{1} = \frac{6}{2}$$

Step 3   Simplify the fraction

$$\frac{\cancel{6}^{3}}{\cancel{2}_{1}} = \frac{3}{1} = 3$$

ACTIVITY 1.13

Complete the following division of fractions:

1 $\frac{1}{7} \div \frac{6}{8} =$ 3 $\frac{4}{5} \div \frac{2}{9} =$ 5 $2\frac{2}{4} \div \frac{3}{5} =$

2 $\frac{2}{9} \div \frac{3}{5} =$ 4 $\frac{2}{4} \div \frac{2}{9} =$

How to multiply and divide fractions by whole numbers

The key to multiplying and dividing fractions by whole numbers is to make the whole number into a fraction. We will look at the process for multiplication first:

Step 1   Place the whole number over 1 to make it into a fraction.

Step 2   Multiply the fraction as before.

Step 3   Simplify the fraction.

WORKED EXAMPLE 1.16

To multiply the following fraction, follow the given steps.

$$\frac{1}{2} \times 4$$

Step 1   Place the whole numbers over 1 to make a fraction

$$\frac{1}{2} \times \frac{4}{1}$$

Step 2   Multiply the fraction straight across

$$\frac{1}{2} \times \frac{4}{1} = \frac{4}{2}$$

Step 3   Simplify the fraction

$$\frac{\cancel{4}^{2}}{\cancel{2}_{1}} = 2$$

Multiply the following fractions by the whole number:

1   $\dfrac{1}{3} \times 5 =$

2   $\dfrac{4}{5} \times 2 =$

3   $\dfrac{1}{10} \times 10 =$

4   $1 \times \dfrac{2}{7} =$

5   $\dfrac{1}{5} \times 3 =$

The process for division is just as straightforward:

Step 1   Place the whole number over 1 to make it into a fraction.

Step 2   Take the second fraction (the one that you are dividing by) and turn it upside down (which turns it into a reciprocal as explained in the section 'How to divide fractions').

Step 3   Multiply the numerator and denominator (as if you are multiplying fractions).

Step 4   Simplify the fraction.

Divide $\dfrac{2}{9}$ by 2.

Step 1   Place the whole number over 1 to make it a fraction

$$\dfrac{2}{9} \div \dfrac{2}{1}$$

Step 2   Take the second fraction you are dividing by and turn it upside down

$$\dfrac{2}{9} \times \left(\dfrac{1}{2}\right) \longleftarrow \text{reciprocal}$$

Step 3   Multiply the numerator and denominator

$$\dfrac{2}{9} \times \dfrac{1}{2} = \dfrac{2}{18}$$

Step 4   Simplify the fraction

$$\dfrac{2^{1}}{18_{9}} = \dfrac{1}{9}$$

ACTIVITY 1.15

Divide the following fractions by whole numbers:

1 $\dfrac{1}{6} \div 2 =$ 4 $\dfrac{4}{5} \div 3 =$

2 $\dfrac{1}{8} \div 5 =$ 5 $\dfrac{7}{8} \div 2 =$

3 $\dfrac{5}{6} \div 2 =$

Cross-cancelling fractions

Cross-cancelling fractions is another way of multiplying fractions, but it can make some very large fractions easier to handle before they are multiplied.

Follow these three steps outlining the cross-cancelling process:

Step 1 Look for a common divisor or multiplication factor between the diagonal numbers, and reduce the fractions.

Step 2 Complete the multiplication as normal.

Step 3 Simplify the fraction.

WORKED EXAMPLE 1.18

$$\frac{81}{21} \times \frac{49}{27}$$

Step 1 Divide the diagonals by the same number (i.e. look for a multiplication factor that is common to both)

Both 21 and 49 can be divided by 7

$$\frac{81}{21_{3}} \xleftarrow{\text{divide by 7}} \frac{49^{7}}{27}$$

$$\frac{81}{3} \times \frac{7}{27}$$

Both 81 and 27 can be divided by 27

$$\frac{\overset{3}{81}}{3} \xrightarrow{\text{divide by 27}} \frac{7}{27_{1}}$$

Step 2 Multiplication

Therefore, the equation has been simplified to

$$\frac{\overset{1}{3}}{\underset{1}{3}} \times \frac{7}{1}$$

Step 3 Simplify the fraction

$$= \frac{7}{1}$$

or 7

Complete the following cross-cancelling and multiplication equations:

1 $\dfrac{7}{20} \times \dfrac{9}{14} =$

2 $\dfrac{8}{12} \times \dfrac{1}{2} =$

3 $\dfrac{6}{12} \times \dfrac{4}{18} =$

4 $\dfrac{5}{10} \times \dfrac{7}{8} =$

5 $\dfrac{13}{14} \times \dfrac{6}{16} =$

Decimals

What are decimals?

The word 'decimal' really means 'based on 10'. We sometimes say 'decimal' when we mean anything to do with our numbering system, but a 'decimal number' usually means there is a decimal point. All numbers may be converted to decimals and fractions. The number to the left of a decimal point is a whole number; the number immediately after the decimal point is a fraction (or part) of 10. So we can write the whole number 4 as the decimal 4.0 (i.e. there are zero extra parts) or as the fraction $\frac{4}{1}$. We can write the number 'one and a half' as the decimal 1.5 or as the mixed number fraction $1\frac{1}{2}$.

How to add decimals

Adding decimals is a very simple process that relies only on knowing how to add. The other major point to avoid errors is to ensure that when you write the numbers you need to add, you follow these basic steps:

Step 1 Write down the numbers, one under the other, with the decimal points lined up.

Step 2 Put in zeros after the decimal point so the numbers have the same length.

Step 3 Add normally, remembering to put the decimal point in the answer. This is easier if you remember to put the decimal point in underneath the numbers you are adding.

WORKED EXAMPLE 1.19

Add 1.464 to 1.5

Line the decimals up	1.464
	+1.5
'Pad' with zeros	1.464
	+1.**500**
Add	1.464
	+1.500
	2.964

ACTIVITY 1.17

Try the following decimal addition questions:

1 $64.752 + 50.5 =$

2 $97.4 + 71.9 =$

3 $3.449 + 1.4 =$

4 $25.3 + 91.7 =$

5 $79.95 + 73.0 =$

How to subtract decimals

Like adding decimals, the process of subtracting decimals is a simple one, relying on the basic concept of subtraction:

Step 1 Write down the two numbers, one under the other, with the decimal points lined up.

Step 2 Add zeros so the numbers have the same length after the decimal point.

Step 3 Subtract normally, remembering to put the decimal point in the answer. This is easier if you remember to put the decimal point in underneath the numbers you are adding.

WORKED EXAMPLE 1.20

Subtract 0.03 from 1.4

Line the decimals up
$$\begin{array}{r} 1.4 \\ -0.03 \end{array}$$

'Pad' with zeros
$$\begin{array}{r} 1.4\mathbf{0} \\ -0.03 \end{array}$$

Subtract
$$\begin{array}{r} 1.40 \\ -0.03 \\ \hline 1.37 \end{array}$$

So, it is just like 140 − 3 = 137, but with the decimal point sitting in its original position. This may be easier if you remember

that you started with a single number that had only one number in front of the decimal space, so our answer will still be the same, especially if we are subtracting such a small amount.

ACTIVITY 1.18

Try the following decimal subtraction questions:

1 14.0 − 4.9 =

2 14.0 − 7.71 =

3 9.9 − 4.0 =

4 12 − 9.13 =

5 16 − 8.1 =

How to multiply decimals

Follow the example given below, tracking it with the steps given:

Step 1 Multiply normally, ignoring the decimal points.

Step 2 Put the decimal point in the answer – it will have as many decimal places as the two original numbers combined.

In other words, just count up how many numbers in total are after the decimal points in both numbers you are multiplying, then the answer should have that many numbers after its decimal point.

Multiply 0.04 by 1.1

start with	0.04×1.1
multiply without decimal points	$4 \times 11 = 44$

0.04 has 2 decimal places and 1.1 has 1 decimal place so the answer has 3 decimal places   0.044

This works because when you multiply without the decimal point, which you do in order to simplify it, we talk about moving the decimal point to the right to get it out of the way. After we move it to the right, and we get the answer, we need to move it back the same number of places, or move it back to the left.

Original   *1 move right*   *2 moves right*   *3 moves right*
0.04×1.1 0.4×1.1 $4. \times 1.1$ $4. \times 11.$
Now to do the multiplication.

$4. \times 11. = 44.$

The next step is to undo the 3 moves to the right with 3 moves to the left.

0.044   0.44   4.4   44.

Try the following questions regarding multiplication of numbers with decimals:

1 $0.7 \times 0.5 =$ 4 $7.49 \times 1000 =$
2 $0.02 \times 0.3 =$ 5 $3.08 \times 10 =$
3 $0.9 \times 0.05 =$

How to divide decimals

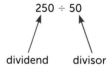

$$250 \div 50$$

dividend   divisor

The number to be divided is called the dividend.

The number which is being used to divide the other number is called the divisor.

$$50\overline{)250}^{\,5}$$

Dividing a decimal number by a whole number

To divide a decimal number by a whole number, use the following steps:

Step 1   Use the long division method (ignoring the decimal point).

Step 2   Then put the decimal point in the same spot as the dividend (the number being divided).

It is worth noting that the answer will always get bigger when you divide by a fraction less than one.

WORKED EXAMPLE 1.22

Divide 0.74 by 2.

Ignore the decimal point and use long division.

Put the decimal point in the answer directly above the decimal point in the dividend.

Step 1   Long division method, ignoring the decimal point

$$0.74 \div 2$$

$$
\begin{array}{r}
37 \\
2\overline{)74} \\
6 \downarrow \\
\hline
14 \\
14 \\
\hline
0
\end{array}
$$

Step 2   We moved the decimal place 2 places to the right to get a whole number, so when we get the answer we need to replace the decimal point by moving it 2 places to the left.

$$37.0$$

The answer is 0.37.

ACTIVITY 1.20

Try the following questions regarding division of numbers with decimals:

1   $0.14 \div 7 =$ 4 $0.20 \div 5 =$

2   $0.63 \div 3 =$ 5 $0.32 \div 8 =$

3   $0.56 \div 2 =$

Dividing by a decimal number

But what if you want to divide by a decimal number?

The trick is to convert the number you are dividing by to a whole number first, by *shifting the decimal point of both numbers to the right*:

$$6.625 \div 0.53 \rightarrow 662.5 \div 53$$

Now you are *dividing by a whole number*, and can continue as normal.

It is safe to do this if you remember to shift the decimal point of *both numbers* the same number of places.

WORKED EXAMPLE 1.23

Divide 1.44 by 0.08

$$1.44 \div 0.08$$

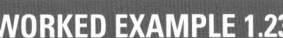

$$1.44 \div 0.08$$

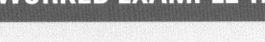

$$= 144 \div 8$$

>>

Step 1   Ignore the decimal point and use long division.

```
      18
   8)144
      8↓
      64
      64
       0
```

The answer is 18.

ACTIVITY 1.21

Try the following questions regarding division of numbers with decimals:

1   1.74 ÷ 0.03 =   4   0.56 ÷ 0.02 =
2   1.16 ÷ 0.02 =   5   0.24 ÷ 0.08 =
3   0.52 ÷ 0.02 =

How to round decimals up or down

Rounding off a decimal is a technique used to limit a result to a manageable size. In practical terms, there is no point working out the answer to a mathematical equation if the answer is much smaller than can be delivered to a client. An example of this is calculating that 1.28678 mL is needed when the syringe can only deliver to one decimal place; that is, it needs to be rounded either up to 1.3 mL or down to 1.2 mL.

We can round to any place. In general, once we decide how many decimal places we are going to use, the number after that decimal place dictates whether the number is moved up to the next number or down to the number below it.

If we were accepting a decimal place to the tenth place (one number to the right of the decimal point), we would need to look at the number that is next to it (in the hundredths column). If this number is 5 or greater, then we would round the number in the tenths column up. If it were below 5, then we would leave it as it is.

WORKED EXAMPLE 1.24

ROUNDING DECIMALS

a   Round 0.64 to the tenths place.

We wish to round 0.64 to the tenths place. That means we only want one digit to appear after the decimal point, so 0.64 will round to 0.6 or 0.7, whichever is closer.

Ones	.	Tenths	Hundredths
0	.	6	4

There is a 4 in the hundredths place. Since this is less than 5, we round down, meaning we leave the 6 in the tenths place and drop the 4 off the end.

The answer is 0.6.

>>

b Round 0.66 to the tenths place.
We wish to round 0.66 to the tenths place. That means we only want one digit to appear after the decimal point, so 0.66 will round to 0.6 or 0.7, whichever is closer.

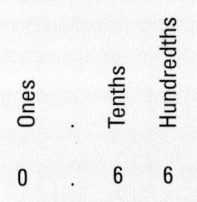

There is a 6 in the hundredths place. Since this is more than 5, we round up, meaning we move the number 6 to 7.
The answer is 0.7.

ACTIVITY 1.22

Round the following examples to the nearest tenth:

1	249.86	4	0.084
2	108.54	5	10.0943
3	0.69		

How to convert decimals to fractions

Decimal numbers are special fractions that have denominators of 10, 100, 1000 or any power of 10. To work out what the denominator is going to be, we need to look at the number of decimal places.

Step 1 Write down the decimal divided by 1.

Step 2 Multiply both top and bottom by 10 for every number to the right of the decimal point. (For example, if there are two numbers after the decimal point, then use 100, if there are three then use 1000, etc.)

Step 3 Simplify the fraction.

Thousands	Hundreds	Tens	Ones	.	Tenths	Hundredths	Thousandths
0	0	2	0	.	6	6	8

WORKED EXAMPLE 1.25

CONVERTING DECIMALS TO FRACTIONS

a Convert 0.25 to a fraction.

An example of this is to convert the decimal 0.25 to a fraction

$\dfrac{0.25}{1}$ multiply both the numerator and denominator by 100, as there are two numbers to the right of the decimal point.

$\dfrac{0.25}{1} \times \dfrac{100}{100}$

>>

>>

$$= \frac{\overset{1}{25}}{\underset{4}{100}}$$ Simplify the fraction by dividing by the largest number in common

$$= \frac{1}{4}$$

b   Convert 0.6 to a fraction.

0.6 has only one decimal place, therefore the denominator of the fraction should be 10:

$$0.6 = \frac{6}{10} \quad \frac{3}{5}$$

c   Convert 0.84 to a fraction.

0.84 has two decimal places, therefore the denominator of the fraction should be 100:

$$0.84 = \frac{84}{100} = \frac{42}{50} = \frac{21}{25}$$

d   Convert 0.668 to a fraction.

0.668 has three decimal places, therefore the denominator of the fraction should be 1000:

$$0.668 = \frac{668}{1000} = \frac{334}{500} = \frac{167}{250}$$

e   Convert 6.4 to a fraction.

6.4 has only one decimal place, therefore the denominator of the fraction should be 10:

$$6.4 = \frac{64}{10} = \frac{32}{5}$$

You can convert this improper fraction to a mixed number:

$$\frac{32}{5} = 6\frac{2}{5}$$

ACTIVITY 1.23

Convert the following decimals to fractions and simplify them:

1   10.137   4   2.15
2   0.933   5   0.6
3   0.24

How to convert fractions to decimals

A fraction, regardless of whether it is an improper or proper fraction, can be made into a decimal by dividing the numerator by the denominator.

Rule: Divide the bottom number into the top number.

(It might be helpful to think of the line in a fraction as a division symbol.)

WORKED EXAMPLE 1.26

EXAMPLE 1

Convert $\frac{27}{10}$ to a decimal.

Divide the denominator into the numerator.

$$
\begin{array}{r}
2.7 \\
10\overline{)27\downarrow} \\
20 \\
\hline
07 \\
\end{array}
$$

Divide 10 into 20
Divide 10 into 7

$= 2.7$

EXAMPLE 2

Convert $\frac{7}{14}$ to a decimal.

Divide the denominator into the numerator

$$
\begin{array}{r}
0.5 \\
14\overline{)7.0} \\
70 \\
\hline
0 \\
\end{array}
$$

Divide 14 into 7. If this does not work, add a decimal point and a zero. Divide 14 into 70. Remember to reinstate the decimal point to your answer after you have solved the equation.

$= 0.5$ 5 becomes 0.5

ACTIVITY 1.24

Change the following fractions into decimals:

1 $\dfrac{115}{25}$ 3 $\dfrac{59}{10}$ 5 $\dfrac{66}{10}$

2 $\dfrac{18}{20}$ 4 $\dfrac{5}{2}$

Ratios and percentages

Ratios and percentages are used throughout society and healthcare on a daily basis. They are a way of expressing 'how many parts' compared to a 'total number of parts'. For example, if there are 20 clients on a hospital ward in total and 10 of them have an infection, then we could express that as a percentage (i.e. 50%) or we could express this as a fraction (i.e. $\frac{10}{20}$ or simplified to $\frac{1}{2}$), or as a ratio (1:2 or 1 in 2 clients have an infection).

Ratios

What are ratios?

Ratios are a way to show the proportion of one part to another part. They are expressed either in numerical format (e.g. 1:5) or in words (e.g. 1 part per five or 1 part to five).

Some drugs have their amount measured in terms of a ratio; for example, adrenaline 1 in 10000 (or 1:10000) is a preparation for injection that contains one part of adrenaline in 10000 parts of this preparation (see Figure 1.7).

This can be confusing for health professionals as the prescribed dose is often given in terms of milligrams, so the ratio must be converted into this form.

Ratios should be reduced to their simplest form, as discussed with fractions (e.g. 2:100 can be simplified to 1:50).

FIGURE 1.7 Drug label – Adrenaline 1 in 10 000

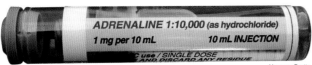

Vanessa Brotto

WORKED EXAMPLE 1.27

STRENGTH AS A RATIO

Adrenaline is an injectable medicine that comes in a 10 mL ampoule containing a '1 in 10 000 solution'.

How do we write this ampoule strength as a ratio?

1:10 000

EXPLANATION

The established method for what this means is that the first part is a weight (i.e. grams is the accepted unit in this situation) and the second part of the phrase is a volume (millilitres). So this means we have 1 g in 10 000 mL in this preparation, which converts to 1000 mg in 10 000 mL, or (by dividing by 1000)

1 mg in 10 mL. If we only have 1 mL of this solution, that means we have much less than 1 g of adrenaline.

Note: *In later sections of this text you will learn how to convert between milligrams and grams and this is required in order to establish how many millilitres of this medicine are required for a prescribed dose.*

Writing ratios in fraction format (and vice versa)

Ratios may be written as a fraction simply by using the first number as the numerator and the second number as the denominator. For example, if a medication is available in a 1:200 strength, this can be expressed as $\frac{1}{200}$.

In order to write fractions in a numerical ratio format, you simply use the numerator as the number on the left and the denominator as the number on the right. For example, $\frac{4}{7}$ can be expressed as a ratio as 4:7.

ACTIVITY 1.25

1 Write the following in a numerical ratio format:

a   1 in 20   d   25 in 100

b   5 parts to 20   e   1 part to 2

c   10 in every 100

>>

>>

2 Write the following ratios in fraction format:

   a 5:10   d 1:10 000

   b 2:4   e 4:5

   c 50:1000

3 Write the following fractions in a numerical ratio format:

   a $\dfrac{1}{4}$ d $\dfrac{3}{4}$

   b $\dfrac{2}{3}$ e $\dfrac{1}{2}$

   c $\dfrac{7}{8}$

Percentages

What are percentages?

'Percentage' is a term that means a part of 100 and it is often referred to using its symbol '%'. There are many medicines that refer to their concentration or strength in percentages, for example, hydrocortisone 0.5% cream (See Figure 1.8). This indicates that 0.5% of the cream contains hydrocortisone. Concentrations and calculating amounts of medicines from percentages is covered in a later chapter.

FIGURE 1.8 Drug label – Hydrocortisone 0.5% cream

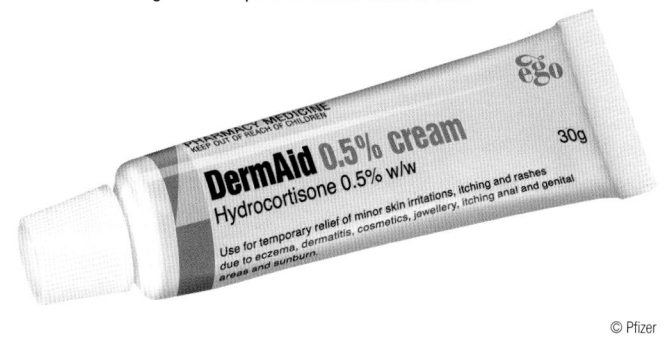

© Pfizer

Percentages are related to ratios and fractions and so they can be converted between these easily; for example, 50% (percentage form) is the same as $\dfrac{50}{100}$ (fraction form), which is the same as 0.5 (decimal form) or 1:2 (ratio form).

Decimals to percentages (and vice versa)

Converting decimals to percentages requires you to *multiply* the decimal number by 100. With a decimal number, this can be easily done by moving the decimal two places to the *right*.

To convert the opposite way (i.e. percentages back into decimals) you need to *divide* the percentage by 100. This can also be done by moving the decimal two places to the *left*.

WORKED EXAMPLE 1.28

DECIMALS TO PERCENTAGES

To convert 0.8 to a percentage we need to multiply by 100.
i.e. $0.8 \times 100 = 80\%$

This could also be done by moving the decimal two places to the right.

0.8

Where there are no other numbers we need to put a zero. Like this:

$0.80 = 80\%$

PERCENTAGES TO DECIMALS

To convert 70% to a decimal we need to divide by 100,
i.e. $70\% \div 100 = 0.7$

This could also be done by moving the decimal two places to the left.

70%   could also be written as 70.0%

$70.0 = 0.70$

1   Convert the following decimals to percentages:
   a   0.17   c   0.5   e   0.9
   b   0.1   d   0.25

2   Convert the following percentages to decimals:
   a   16%   c   55%   e   98%
   b   22%   d   0.05%

Fractions to percentages (and vice versa)

Converting fractions to percentages requires you to *multiply* the fraction by 100.

To convert the opposite way (i.e. percentages back into fractions) you need to *divide* the percentage by 100.

WORKED EXAMPLE 1.29

FRACTIONS TO PERCENTAGES

To convert $\frac{4}{5}$ to a percentage, we need to multiply by 100.

$$\frac{4}{5} \times 100$$

$$\frac{4}{5} \times \frac{100}{1} = 80\%$$

\>\>

>>

To do this you can also do the following.

$4 \div 5 \times 100 = 80\%$

PERCENTAGES TO FRACTIONS

To convert 75% to a fraction we need to divide by 100.

$$75\% \div 100 = \frac{75}{100}$$

Remember that percentages are always numbers shown as a part of 100, so in fraction form the percentage number goes on top of 100.

ACTIVITY 1.27

1 Convert the following fractions to percentages:

a $\dfrac{2}{10}$

d $\dfrac{7}{25}$

b $\dfrac{25}{50}$

e $\dfrac{8}{10}$

c $\dfrac{3}{4}$

2 Convert the following percentages to fractions:

a 18%

d 94%

b 28%

e 0.02%

c 57%

Proportions

What are proportions?

'Proportion' is a term used in mathematics to indicate that one fraction, ratio or percentage is equivalent or 'in proportion to' another. In the true sense of the word, 'proportion' relates to the amount of something that is part of a whole. This forms the basis for the proportions approach to solving dosage calculations. If performed correctly according to the rules described in the following chapters, it is one of the simplest ways of approaching dosage calculations without needing to remember complex formulae and how to apply them.

There are a number of ways of writing proportion equations, usually as either ratios or fractions. They have the same meaning; that is, to show that one ratio or fraction is equivalent or equal to the other. The following text illustrates the two methods that may be used, but remember, they mean the same thing. The only rule is that you must always have the equivalent unit on the same side of the equals sign (i.e. mg is on the same side of the equals sign for both equations, as illustrated on the following page). It does not matter which side you choose for mg or mL as long as you are consistent for both equations. You could not have one equation with mg on the left and the other with mg on the right – you must be consistent with how you set out the equations.

PROPORTIONS

Proportions MUST always be consistent with the value you place on each side of the equals sign.

Proportion written as a ratio: 50 mg : 100 mL = 1 mg : 2 mL (meaning a ratio of 50 mg to 100 mL is the same as a ratio of 1 mg to 2 mL).

Proportion written as a fraction: $\dfrac{50\ mg}{100\ mL} = \dfrac{1\ mg}{2\ mL}$

Rather than writing these two proportions side by side, we can separate them onto two lines as two equations to make it easier to understand:

Equation 1:

$$\frac{50\ mg}{100\ mL}$$

is the same as writing
50 mg : 100 mL
which is the same as writing
50 mg = 100 mL

Equation 2:

$$\frac{1\ mg}{2\ mL}$$

is the same as writing
1 mg : 2 mL
which is the same as writing
1 mg = 2 mL

We can solve dosage calculations using a proportions approach if we know three of the values in the proportion (i.e. there is only one unknown value).

WORKED EXAMPLE 1.30

SOLVING PROPORTIONS WHERE ONE VALUE IS UNKNOWN

An example here is how we refer to the proportion as an amount of medication in relation to the total amount available in a bottle. So if a medication bottle contains 250 mg/5 mL and you want 500 mg, then you structure the proportion as follows:

Equation 1:

250 mg/5 mL

is the same as writing

250 mg : 5 mL

which is the same as writing

250 mg = 5 mL

>>

Equation 2: We only know the mg part of this equation so this is written as

500 mg = x mL

We need to use the rules we have learnt about mathematics in this chapter if we want to solve for the missing value (an x is used traditionally but you can use any symbol you like for this).

If we have (in the
medication bottle): 250 mg = 5 mL

Then we want: 500 mg = x mL

| Ensure you put the same units on the same side of the equation (i.e. here both equations have mg on the left side). |

Cross-multiply: 250 mg = 5 mL

500 mg = x mL

| Multiply everything diagonally (i.e. 250 × x = 250x and 500 × 5 = 2500). |

So: $250x = 2500$

Solve for x: $\dfrac{250x}{250} = \dfrac{2500}{250}$

| Divide both sides by 250 in order to get x by itself. |

x = 10 mL of this solution contains 500 mg of medication

So the whole proportion may be said that if 250 mg = 5 mL, then the equivalent is 500 mg = 10 mL.

2 UNITS OF MEASUREMENT

Introduction

Healthcare professionals need to have a good understanding of the different units that are used in healthcare and a strong ability to convert between these units (e.g. convert from milligrams [mg] to grams [g]). They also need to know the symbols and abbreviations for each unit, as there have been many documented fatalities in Australia and New Zealand where one unit was mistaken for another on a medication chart, resulting in clients receiving overdoses (some were overdosed 1000 times the prescribed dose when the symbol for micrograms was confused with milligrams!).

Throughout most of the world (although not the United States of America), the International System of Units (SI) (based on the metric system) is used in society, especially in science and medicine. There are two other systems of measurement that are not used in healthcare in Australia or New Zealand; these are the apothecary and the household systems. Both of these are predominantly used in healthcare in the US and in non-scientific areas in other parts of the world.

This chapter briefly introduces the three common systems of measurement seen in healthcare but focuses on the SI system of units (metric) that is used in Australia and New Zealand. These metric units are explained, and converting between units is also covered.

Systems of measurement: an overview

The household system of units

The household system does not have an exact or internationally recognised set of standards for measurement. Typical measures that are used in this system are *teaspoon*, *tablespoon*, *cup*, *quart*, etc. Technically, it is easy to convert from this system to metric (e.g. one cup usually contains between 230 and 250 mL) but, as there is no exact approved standard, this does vary. Hence, it is easy to understand why it may be risky to use this system of measurement when administering medicines to clients. Medicines used to be administered to children using the *teaspoon* measure until it became apparent that a teaspoon from one cutlery set could vary as much as 5 mL from another teaspoon and that could be an overdose in paediatric medicines.

The apothecary system of units

The apothecary system of measurement has a long history from its origins in ancient Greece. As a whole, it is not well known in contemporary Australian and New Zealand societies, although some units of this system may be well recognised (i.e. Roman numerals [I, II, III, IV, etc.]). This system may be recognisable to healthcare professionals as the system used for the number of tablets to be given to a client on a medication chart, although these symbols are no longer accepted units for medication charts in Australia (see **Figure 2.1**). These abbreviations are said to be 'error-prone' and are not best practice (as they are easily misinterpreted, leading to errors); however, many prescribers still use these symbols and, though not legally accepted, they are still found on some medication charts. The other common units from this system include *grains*, *ounces*, *pints* and *gallons*.

FIGURE 2.1 Diagram of apothecary measurements often still found on medication charts

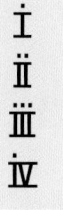

The metric system/International System of Units

The 'metric system' is a system of measurement that is focused in general terms around a single unit known as a 'metre'. This system is used internationally and is the basis for the 'SI units' also known as the 'International System of Units'. It is based on the number 10 and so can be called a 'decimal system', and it centres upon seven 'base units'. Not all of these units are applicable in healthcare; those that are commonly used in dosage calculations include *metres*, *grams*, *litres* and *moles*.

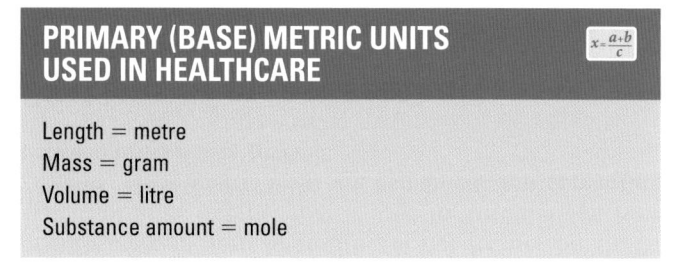

PRIMARY (BASE) METRIC UNITS USED IN HEALTHCARE

$$x = \frac{a+b}{c}$$

Length = metre
Mass = gram
Volume = litre
Substance amount = mole

The metric system is preferred as the system to use when prescribing and giving medicines (even in the US). It is recognised as a reliable system of measurement that is accurate and relatively easy to use in healthcare.

Metric prefixes

The base units (metre, gram, litre, moles) are given prefixes to illustrate the proportion of that base unit (e.g. one milligram is one-thousandth of one gram). The most common metric prefixes used in healthcare include *kilo-*, *milli-* and *micro-*. They are combined with the base units (e.g. kilometre, millilitre, microgram).

METRIC PREFIXES

$x = \frac{a+b}{c}$

micro = one-millionth or 0.000 001 or $\frac{1}{1000000}$ of the base unit

milli = one-thousandth or 0.001 or $\frac{1}{1000}$ of the base unit

centi = one-hundredth or 0.01 or $\frac{1}{100}$ of the base unit

deci = one-tenth or 0.1 or $\frac{1}{10}$ of the base unit

kilo = one thousand or 1000 times the base unit

Most metric prefixes are easily converted between steps by multiplying or dividing by 1000 (i.e. to go to a smaller unit you would *multiply* the figure by 1000 but to go up to a larger unit you would *divide* the figure by 1000). For example, if you wanted to convert 3 milligrams to micrograms (i.e. move to a smaller unit), you would multiply 3 milligrams by 1000, giving a total of 3000 micrograms. If you wanted to convert 500 milligrams to grams (i.e. move to a larger unit), you would divide by 1000, giving a total of 0.5 grams. The only prefixes that do not fit in this way are *centi-* (one-hundredth) and *deci-* (one-tenth).

Metric abbreviations

Each unit in the metric system has been given an abbreviation within the SI unit standards. Some of these units have more than one abbreviation, which can cause confusion (e.g. micrograms may be abbreviated as µg, mcg or microg and the confusion this has caused on medication charts has resulted in client deaths when mg is mistaken for µg). It is for this reason that the Australian Commission on Safety and Quality in Health Care released a set of national guidelines for abbreviations to be used in medication charts. It recommended that micrograms be written on medication charts in full or using the abbreviation 'microg' to reduce any possible confusion.

Table 2.1 shows the common SI units used in healthcare alongside their SI abbreviation. Note that lower-case and upper-case characters must be written exactly as shown in this table. A common mistake is writing 'ml' or 'mls' instead of the standard official unit abbreviation, which is 'mL', and this can lead to medication errors. A noted exception to this is the abbreviation for 'litre', which is technically 'l'; however, given this can be mistaken for the number '1' it is often written in upper-case 'L'.

TABLE 2.1 SI metric system

	Unit	Abbreviation	Equivalents
Mass	**gram** (base unit)	g	1 g = 1000 mg = 1000 000 microg
	milligram	mg	0.001 g = 1 mg = 1000 microg
	microgram	microg	0.000001 g = 0.001 mg = 1 microg
	kilogram	kg	1 kg = 1000 g
Amount of substance (particles or elementary entities)	**Mole** (base unit)	mol	1 mol = 1000 mmol
	millimole	mmol	0.001 mol = 1 mmol
Volume	**litre** (base unit)	L	1 L = 1000 mL
	millilitre	mL	0.001 L = 1 mL
Length	**metre** (base unit)	m	1 m = 100 cm = 1000 mm
	centimetre	cm	0.01 m = 1 cm = 10 mm
	millimetre	mm	0.001 m = 0.1 cm = 1 mm

Other units seen in healthcare: units, moles and millimoles

Units

Some medications have their amount measured in 'units'. This can be confusing as the term 'units' here is being used as the actual unit of measurement. Common medicines that have their amount described in this way are insulin and heparin (see Figures 2.2 and 2.3).

Health professionals do not usually need to convert from these 'units' into another form of measurement (as there are no equivalents in grams, etc.) but they *do* need to calculate doses. In this instance, the dosage calculation is done exactly the same way as any other dosage calculation – the type of unit does not affect this.

The word 'unit' should be written in full to avoid confusion. In the past, the symbol 'U' was accepted but that tragically resulted in a number of adverse events with clients receiving overdoses of insulin (e.g. when '10U Insulin' was misread as '100' and the client received 10 times the intended dose of insulin).

FIGURE 2.2 Infusion label – Heparin 25 000 units

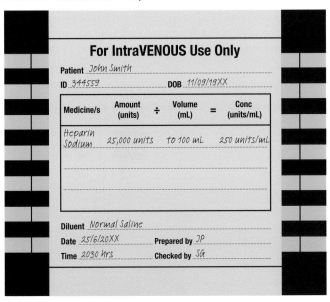

For IntraVENOUS Use Only

Patient _John Smith_
ID _344559_   DOB _11/09/19XX_

Medicine/s	Amount (units)	÷	Volume (mL)	=	Conc (units/mL)
Heparin Sodium	25,000 units		to 100 mL		250 units/mL

Diluent _Normal Saline_
Date _25/6/20XX_   Prepared by _JP_
Time _2030 hrs_   Checked by _SG_

FIGURE 2.3 Infusion label – Actrapid in units

For IntraVENOUS Use Only

Patient _John Smith_
ID _344559_   DOB _11/09/19XX_

Medicine/s	Amount (units)	÷	Volume (mL)	=	Conc (units/mL)
Actrapid	100 units		to 100 mL		1 unit/mL

Diluent _Normal Saline_
Date _26/4/20XX_   Prepared by _JP_
Time _2045 hrs_   Checked by _SG_

Moles and millimoles

A mole is an SI unit of measurement commonly referred to in chemistry where it is the amount of a substance. One mole should contain 6.02×10^{23} particles or 'elementary entities'. Moles are a convenient unit that make descriptions simpler rather than performing calculations involving very large exponential numbers, such as multiples of 6.02×10^{23}! Healthcare professionals are not usually required to convert between moles and millimoles and the other SI units; however, there are a few medicines that use millimoles as their units (e.g. potassium chloride comes in a 10 mmol/100 mL preparation – see Figure 2.4).

FIGURE 2.4 Potassium 10 mmol in 100 mL infusion bag

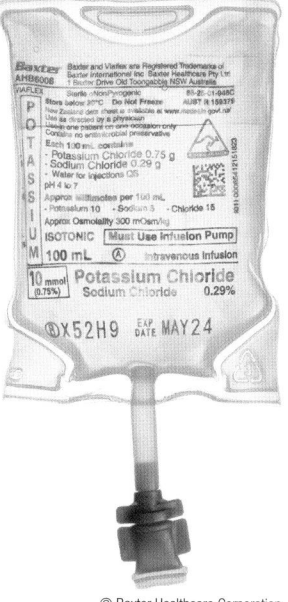

© Baxter Healthcare Corporation

Reducing risk to clients concerning units of measurement

It has already been explained in this chapter that clients have died from health professionals mistakenly converting between units and overdosing the client. There have also been numerous fatalities linked to unclear or illegible medication orders on charts. Health professionals should remember this and follow the '10 rules for accurate written and interpretation of metric notation' outlined below concerning units of measurement and medication administration.

10 RULES FOR ACCURATE WRITTEN AND INTERPRETATION OF METRIC NOTATION

Rule 1 The unit or abbreviation always follows the amount (e.g. 5 g not g 5).

Rule 2 Do not put a full stop after the unit abbreviation because it may be mistaken for the number 1 if poorly written (e.g. mg not mg.).

Rule 3 Do not add an 's' to make the unit plural because it may be misread for another unit (e.g. mL not mLs).

Rule 4 Separate the amount from the unit so the number and unit of measure do not run together because the unit can be mistaken as zero or zeros, risking a 10-fold or 100-fold overdose (e.g. 20 mg not 20mg).

Rule 5 Place thin spaces for amounts at or above 10 000 (e.g. 10 000 microg not 10000 microg).

Rule 6 Decimals are used to designate fractional amounts (e.g. 1.5 mL not $1\frac{1}{2}$ mL).

Rule 7 Use a leading zero to emphasise the decimal point for fractional amounts less than 1. Without the zero, the amount may be interpreted as a whole number, resulting in serious overdosing (e.g. 0.5 mg not .5 mg).

>>

Rule 8 Omit unnecessary or trailing zeros that can be misread as part of the amount if the decimal point is not seen (e.g. 1.5 mg not 1.50 mg).

Rule 9 Do not use the abbreviation μg for microgram because it might be mistaken for mg, which is 1000 times the intended amount (e.g. 150 microg not 150 μg or 150 mcg).

Rule 10 Do not use the abbreviation cc for mL because the unit can be mistaken for zeros (e.g. 500 mL not 500 cc).

Always ask the prescriber to clarify if you are not sure of the abbreviation or notation used. Never guess!

Measuring solids

Medications are often in solid forms such as powders, tablets and granules. When we discuss the 'amount' of a solid medication we often refer to it as the 'mass' or 'weight'. The National Physical Laboratory (2010) in the United Kingdom explains that, though mass and weight are terms that are often used interchangeably, mass is the 'amount of material in an object' while weight is the 'gravitational force acting on a body'. These terms are technically different in scientific terms but are often used to describe the mass.

Converting between metric units

Earlier in this chapter we explained that to convert to a smaller unit you would multiply the figure by 1000, and to change to a larger unit you would divide the figure by 1000 (an exception was for *centi-* and *deci-*). The most important thing for a health professional to remember is the order of the metric prefixes to know how many times you need to divide or multiply by 1000. Table 2.2 shows the order of the prefixes and their equivalent value to the base unit (gram, litre, metre, mole).

Converting micrograms into milligrams (and vice versa)

Since a *micro*gram is 1000 times smaller than a *milli*gram, to convert an amount from micrograms to milligrams we need to *divide* by 1000.

TABLE 2.2 Relationship and value of metric units, with comparison of common metric units used in healthcare

Prefix	KILO-	Hecto-	Deca-	BASE	DECI-	CENTI-	MILLI-	Decimilli-	Centimilli-	MICRO-
Value to base	1000	100	10	1	0.1	0.01	0.001	0.0001	0.00001	0.000001
Weight	kilogram			gram			milligram			microgram
Volume				litre	decilitre		millilitre			
Length				metre		centimetre	millimetre			

CHAPTER 2

WORKED EXAMPLE 2.1

Convert 500 micrograms to milligrams.

500 micrograms *divided* by 1000 = 0.5 milligrams

This could also be done by moving the decimal place three spaces to the left and adding a leading zero before the decimal point.

500. micrograms = 0.500 milligrams = 0.5 milligrams

SAFETY ⚠️

Notice that converting 500 microg to mg results in a decimal fraction that is less than 1. For safety, always place a zero to the left of the decimal point to emphasise any decimal number that has a value less than 1.

The opposite is the case if we want to convert an amount from milligrams to micrograms – we *multiply* by 1000.

Notice that to multiply a number by 1000 using the shortcut, you are moving the decimal point three places to the right. Sometimes to complete this operation, you need to add zeros to hold the places equal to the number of zeros in the equivalent (e.g. if you are changing 2 mg to microg, you need to add three zeros [i.e. 2.000] to have three places to the right of the decimal point).

The same principles apply for converting from microlitres into millilitres and millilitres to microlitres, although these are not common conversions in healthcare.

RULE $x = \frac{a+b}{c}$

To convert from a smaller to a larger unit of measurement, divide by the conversion factor.

THINK: *Smaller* is going up to *larger*, so you will divide.

Smaller ↑ Larger → Divide (÷)

Converting milligrams into grams (and vice versa)

Since a milligram is 1000 times smaller than a gram, to convert an amount from milligrams to grams we need to *divide* by 1000.

WORKED EXAMPLE 2.2

Convert 800 milligrams to grams.

800 milligrams *divided* by 1000 = 0.8 grams

This could also be done by moving the decimal place three spaces to the left.

800. milligrams = 0.800 grams = 0.8 grams

The opposite is the case if we want to convert an amount from grams to milligrams – we *multiply* by 1000.

The same principles apply for converting between millilitres and litres, which are common conversions in healthcare.

Converting grams into kilograms (and vice versa)

Since a gram is 1000 times smaller than a kilogram, to convert an amount from grams to kilograms we need to *divide* by 1000.

WORKED EXAMPLE 2.3

Convert 2 grams to kilograms.

    2 grams *divided* by 1000 = 0.002 kilograms

    This could also be done by moving the decimal place three spaces to the left.

    2 grams = 002.0 grams = 0.002 kilograms

The opposite is the case if we want to convert an amount from kilograms to grams – we *multiply* by 1000.

The same principles apply for converting between litres and kilolitres, although this is not common in healthcare.

Converting grams into micrograms (and vice versa)

Since a microgram is 1 000 000 times smaller than a gram, to convert an amount from grams to micrograms we need to multiply by 1 000 000. This can also be done by first converting grams into milligrams (*multiply* by 1000) and then converting milligrams into micrograms (*multiply again* by 1000).

WORKED EXAMPLE 2.4

Convert 0.2 gram to micrograms.

    0.2 g *multiplied* by 1 000 000 = 200 000 microg

    This could also be done by moving the decimal place six spaces to the right.

    0.2 gram = 0.200 000 grams = 200 000 micrograms

RULE

To convert from a larger to a smaller unit of measurement, multiply by the conversion factor.

THINK: *Larger* is going down to *smaller*, so you will multiply.

    Larger ↓ Smaller → Multiply (×)

The opposite is the case if we want to convert an amount from micrograms to grams – we *divide* by 1 000 000. This can also be done by first converting micrograms into milligrams (*divide* by 1000) and then converting milligrams into grams (*divide again* by 1000).

The same principles apply for converting between litres and microlitres, although this is not common in healthcare.

MATHS TIP

$x = \dfrac{a+b}{c}$

Remember this diagram when converting dosages within the metric system.

Move decimal point three places to the left for each step.

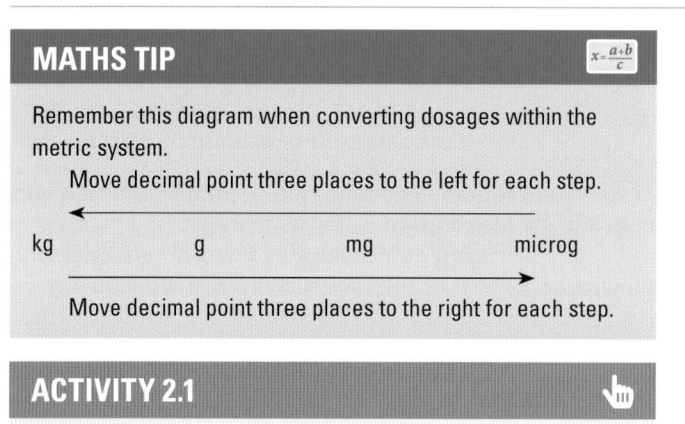

kg   g   mg   microg

Move decimal point three places to the right for each step.

ACTIVITY 2.1

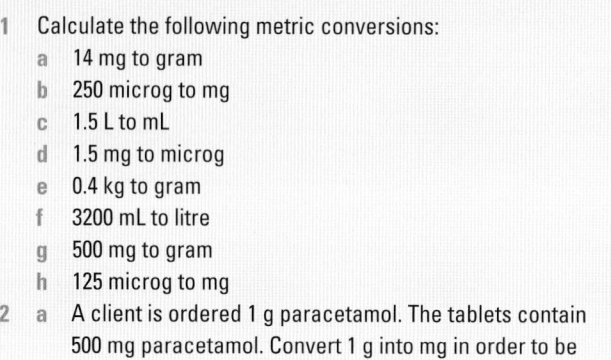

1   Calculate the following metric conversions:
   a   14 mg to gram
   b   250 microg to mg
   c   1.5 L to mL
   d   1.5 mg to microg
   e   0.4 kg to gram
   f   3200 mL to litre
   g   500 mg to gram
   h   125 microg to mg

2   a   A client is ordered 1 g paracetamol. The tablets contain 500 mg paracetamol. Convert 1 g into mg in order to be able to calculate the number of tablets required.

   b   A client is ordered 0.5 g ampicillin. The capsules contain 250 mg ampicillin. Convert 0.5 g into mg in order to calculate the number of capsules.

   c   A client is ordered 0.125 mg of digoxin. The tablets contain 62.5 microg digoxin. Convert 0.125 mg into microg in order to be able to calculate the number of tablets.

   d   A client is ordered 1.2 g lithium carbonate. The tablets contain 400 mg lithium. Convert 1.2 g into mg in order to be able to calculate the number of tablets.

   e   A client has drunk a 1.25 L bottle of soft drink this morning and you need to document it on their fluid balance chart in mL. Convert 1.25 L into mL.

3   a   There are _____ mg in 1.2 g.
   b   There are _____ mg in 0.7 g.
   c   There are _____ microg in 0.05 mg.
   d   There are _____ microg in 2.3 mg.
   e   There are _____ microg in 1.07 g.
   f   There are _____ mg in 1.4 kg.
   g   Which is smaller? 62 microg or 0.006 mg
   h   Which is smaller? 600 microg or 0.06 mg
   i   Which is smaller? 6 microg or 0.6 mg
   j   Which is smaller? 6 microg or 0.0006 mg

Measuring liquids

Liquids can be measured in a variety of ways in healthcare; each method has its benefits and risks in terms of ease of use and accuracy. Graduated spoons and droppers may sometimes be used but these are often questionable in terms of accuracy. The more common methods used to measure liquids in healthcare involve measuring cups/jugs and syringes.

Measuring cup or jug

A measuring cup or jug is usually a transparent container that has graduations of volume marked on the side. It allows the user to pour a liquid into the container and be able to see approximately how much liquid is in the container.

These measuring cups and jugs are good for approximate amounts but are notoriously inaccurate and sometimes dangerous to use in medication administration (especially with small volumes or potent medicines).

When a liquid is poured into the container, the user needs to hold the container up to be in line with their eyes to avoid misreading the amount in the container. This is due to a 'parallax error', which can cause the user to overestimate the amount of liquid in the cup if they look *down* at the container, or underestimate the amount of liquid if they look *up* at the container (see Figure 2.5). Therefore, the only way to find the true amount of liquid in a measuring cup (i.e. medicine cup) is to look at the fluid line exactly at eye level.

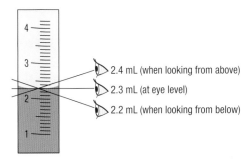

FIGURE 2.5 Parallax error

2.4 mL (when looking from above)
2.3 mL (at eye level)
2.2 mL (when looking from below)

The meniscus is a concave (curved) shape that may be visible when the measuring cup is held to the user's eye level – it is caused by the surface tension of the liquid being drawn up the sides of the measuring container (see Figure 2.6). When assessing for the amount of liquid in a measuring cup or jug, the user should take the reading from the base of the meniscus (if visible).

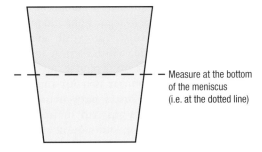

FIGURE 2.6 Meniscus and point of measurement in a medicine cup

Measure at the bottom of the meniscus (i.e. at the dotted line)

It is also important to note that health professionals should try to pour away from the medication label (i.e. pour with the bottle label facing uppermost) as this can prevent spilt drips of the medicine running over the label, which can mask important information.

Syringe

A syringe is superior to a measuring cup or jug in terms of volume accuracy with liquid medicines. These are also usually transparent, with graduations of volume marked along the syringe barrel. Syringes need to draw the fluid up (pulling the plunger away from the barrel) in order to allow the fluid to enter the syringe.

There are numerous types and sizes of syringes and most of these are beyond the scope of this chapter; however, it is important that the health professional uses the smallest appropriate-sized syringe to draw up the liquid in order to ensure the best accuracy (e.g. use a 1 mL syringe to draw up 0.5 mL of fluid as the graduations allow easy reading of the volume in the syringe compared with using a 20 mL syringe to draw up 0.5 mL, where the graduations on this syringe would not allow the user to measure this amount accurately).

The volume in the syringe is read from the upper black ring of the plunger, not the lower black ring; this can be seen in Figures 2.7 and 2.8.

FIGURE 2.7 2 mL syringe with needle unit measuring 1 mL

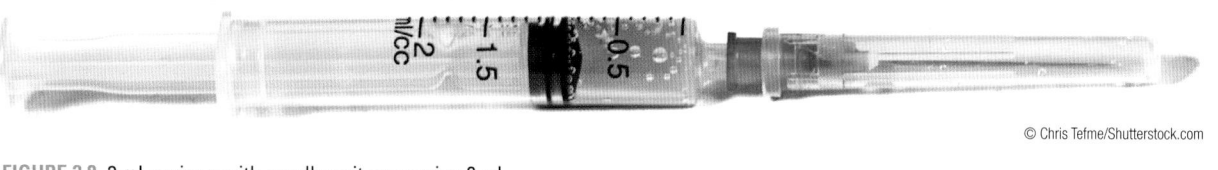

© Chris Tefme/Shutterstock.com

FIGURE 2.8 3 mL syringe with needle unit measuring 2 mL

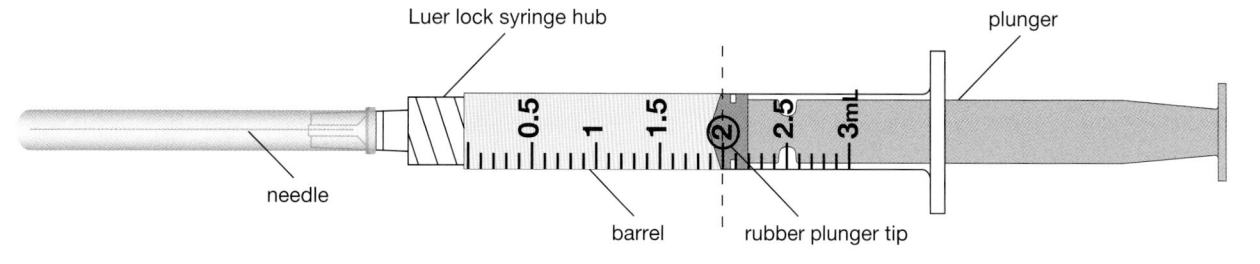

Some syringes are measured in millilitres and others are measured in 'units' (the ones in units are often used for heparin or insulin doses, which are also expressed in 'units' rather than the standard units) (see Figures 2.9(a) and 2.9(b)).

FIGURE 2.9(a) Standard U-100 insulin syringe

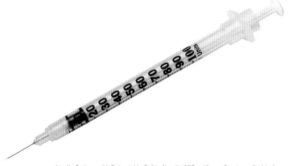

Insulin Syringe with Retractable Safety Needle 27G x 13mm. Courtesy of mldevices

FIGURE 2.9(b) Example of a Lo-Dose insulin syringe

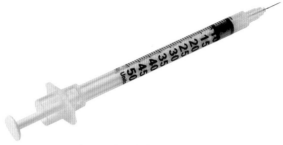

Insulin Syringe with Retractable Safety Needle 29G x 8mm. Courtesy of mldevices

ACTIVITY 2.2

1   Draw a line to indicate where you would draw the liquid up to with these syringes:

a   Administer 0.75 mL

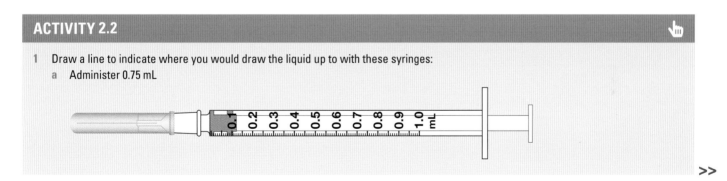

>>

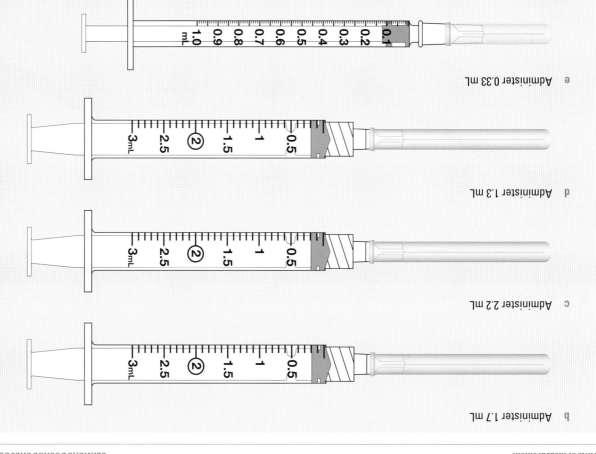

b   Administer 1.7 mL

c   Administer 2.2 mL

d   Administer 1.3 mL

e   Administer 0.33 mL

f   Administer 65 units of insulin

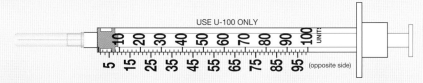

g   Administer 27 units of insulin

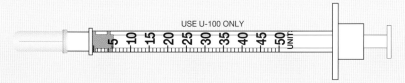

h   Administer 75 units of insulin

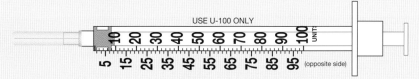

i   Administer 4.4 mL

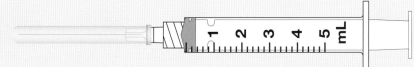

>>

j   Administer 16 mL

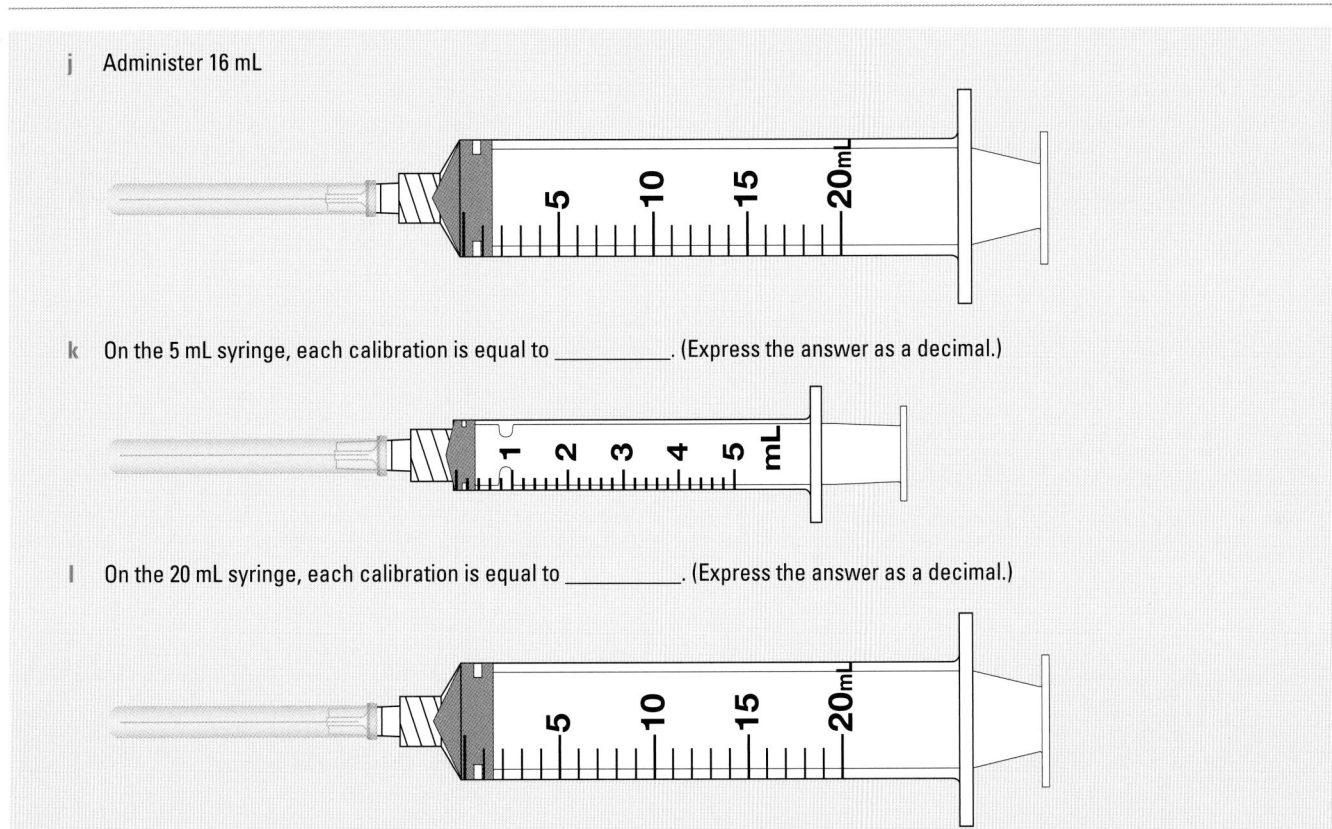

k   On the 5 mL syringe, each calibration is equal to _____ . (Express the answer as a decimal.)

l   On the 20 mL syringe, each calibration is equal to _____ . (Express the answer as a decimal.)

m On the 10 mL syringe, each calibration is equal to _____. (Express the answer as a decimal.)

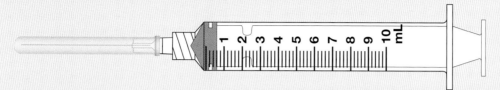

2 Draw a fluid level inside these medicine cups to indicate the following doses:

a 2.5 mL

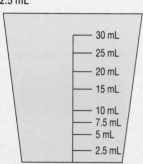

b 12.5 mL

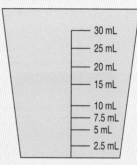

>>

>>

3 What is the volume of liquid found in each of these measuring devices?

a Medicine cup with …..

b Medicine cup with …..

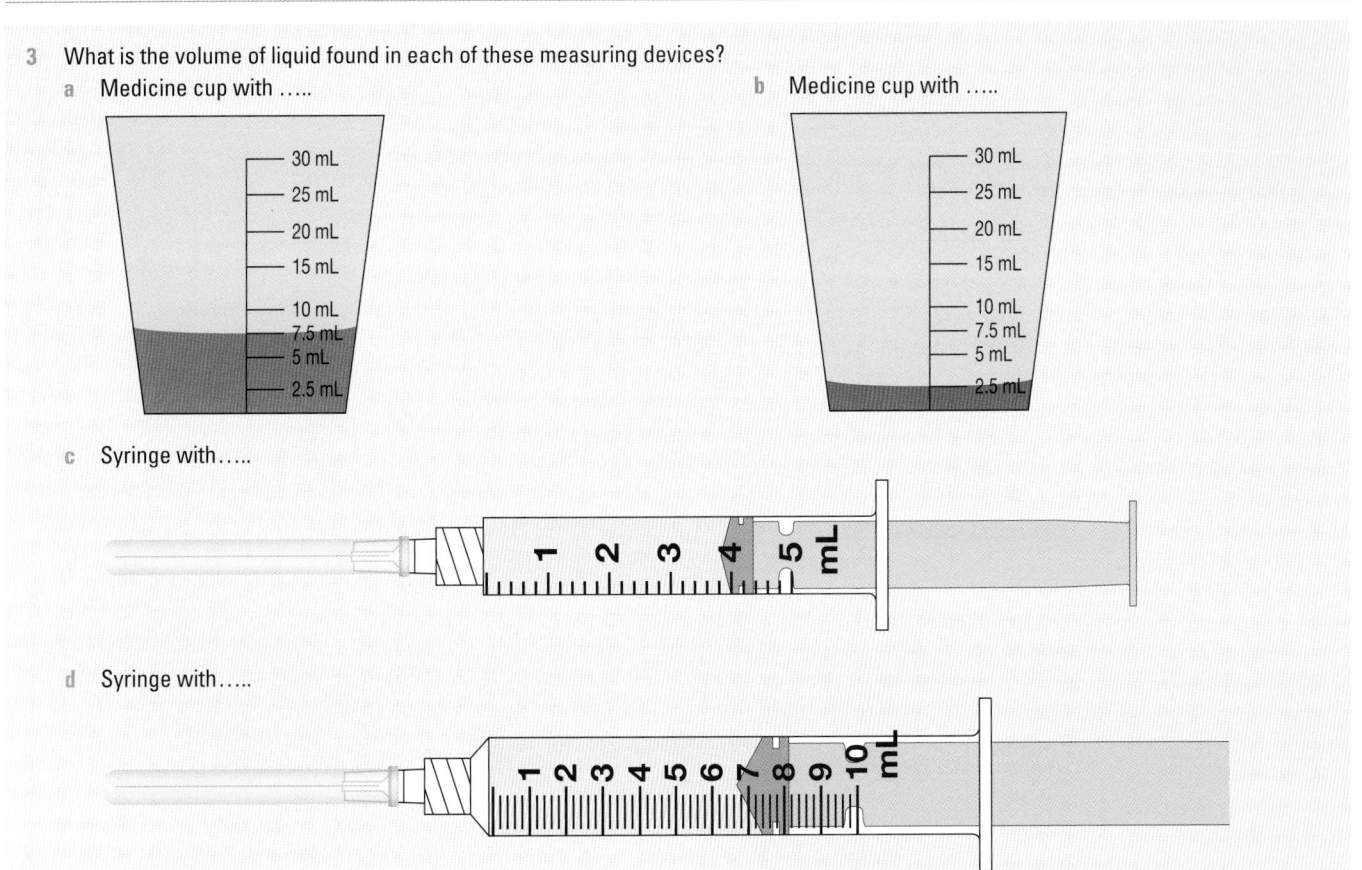

c Syringe with…..

d Syringe with…..

3 MEDICATION CHARTS

Introduction

Correct interpretation of a medication chart is one of the most important steps in the delivery of medicines to a client. There are several parts to a medication order that have to be checked in every situation in order to prevent a potentially lethal drug error.

It is the responsibility of any healthcare professional who is administering medicine to a client to ensure a number of points.

The healthcare professional must:

- be able to read the order and interpret it correctly
- be able to identify the correct medicine
- be able to prepare the correct dosage of the medicine
- be able to comprehend the legal and ethical implications when administering medicine to clients
- ensure they can identify:
  - the correct route for the medicine to be given
  - the correct client for it to be given to
  - the correct time for it to be given.

This chapter looks specifically at the National Inpatient Medication Chart (NIMC) and the National Residential Medication Chart (NRMC) designed by the Australian Commission on Safety and Quality in Health Care, as well as the National Medication Chart developed by the Safe Medication Management Programme for the Health Quality & Safety Commission New Zealand. These medication charts were designed to focus on reducing medication errors within all Australian and New Zealand healthcare settings. Some important features of these charts have been included in this chapter and further content is available online.

Inpatient charts used in Australia and New Zealand

The Australian Commission on Safety and Quality in Health Care and the New Zealand Health Quality & Safety Commission have designed separate national inpatient medication charts

(NIMC) and residential medication charts (NRMC) that are intended to reduce the incidence of medication errors in the ordering and administration of medicines.

Medication errors are the cause of a number of disabilities and deaths across healthcare agencies in both countries. The national medication charts aim to reduce the number of errors that are made by addressing the cause of errors in prescribing, dispensing and administering medicine.

The NRMC was developed to evidence best practice and be compliant with accreditation standards, expected outcomes and the *Aged Care Act 1997*. It aims to improve the safety of medication management in residential aged care facilities (RACFs) in Australia through standardised medication charting and medication management practice.

The residential medication chart enables the direct supply by a pharmacy of many PBS/RPBS and non-PBS medicines without the need for the traditional paper-based prescription. Once the prescriber has filled in all sections of the residential chart, it may be photocopied, faxed or scanned and emailed to the pharmacy for filling of the prescription. The prescription may also be written digitally via an electronic medication chart. Whenever there is any change to the chart, a full copy of the chart must be included with the new order.

The residential medication chart is a wide-ranging document that is explained more fully in Chapter 10.

The legality of the medication chart

There are a number of factors that need to be present for the medication chart to be considered best practice and meet relevant legal requirements.

When looking at the identification part of the inpatient medication chart, there needs to be either a current identification label for that client on the medication chart or at least three identifiers – such as the client's name, unit record (UR) number and date of birth – written in the identification box (see Figure 3.1). The residential chart stipulates that the identification panel must contain *at least* the resident's full name, date of birth and residential aged care identification number (RACS ID), as this stands for the resident's address. If these areas are not completed, then the medication chart is non-valid and therefore cannot be used. It is the prescriber of the medication who must fill in the client identifiers. This is to prevent the medication chart being labelled for the wrong client.

Following the guidelines, each order also needs to include all the elements needed to give a medicine. These elements are:

- the date the medicine was ordered
- the administration times
- the route for administration of the medicine
- the frequency of administration
- the dose ordered
- the generic name of the medicine (preferred)
- the indication for the medicine (for PRN medicines only in NZ)

- the prescriber's signature and their surname printed (prescriber's signature only in NZ, but prescribers must complete the sample signature section)
- the contact number for the prescriber (preferred in NZ; registration number required in sample signature section).

FIGURE 3.1 Client identification labels (a) Client identification label (Australian) (b) NRMC client identification label

(a) Affix patient identification label here

URN:	
Family name:	Not a valid prescription unless identifiers present
Given names:	
Address:	
Date of birth:	**Sex:** ☐ M ☐ F

First prescriber to print patient name and check label correct: ....

(b)

Personal Particulars		ALERT
Resident Name		Resident with similar name? Yes / No
Resident Preferred Name	Age	URN / MRN No.
Date of Birth	Gender M / F	Date of Photo ➝
IHI	Room No.	RAC ID

1

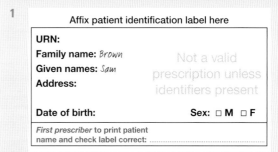

Affix patient identification label here

URN:	
Family name: *Brown*	Not a valid prescription unless identifiers present
Given names: *Sam*	
Address:	
Date of birth:	**Sex:** ☐ M ☐ F

First prescriber to print patient name and check label correct: ....

In your hospital ward, you have a client by the name of Samantha Brown. She is a 35-year-old female who has been admitted for reconstruction of the left shoulder. Dr Gray, thinking that someone would place an ID label over the name, has left the name written as Sam Brown.

In a room further down the ward, a 63-year-old male client by the name of Samuel Brown has been admitted for stabilisation of his atrial fibrillation. He has a history of hypertension and has type 2 diabetes.

Using this example, write down some of the ramifications of having Samantha Brown's medication chart wrongly labelled as Samuel Brown. Fill in the client identification details that would have prevented this error.

>>

Affix patient identification label here

2

URN:

Family name: *Maher*

Given names: *Chris*

Address:

Not a valid
prescription unless
identifiers present

Date of birth: **Sex:** □ **M** □ **F**

First prescriber to print patient
name and check label correct: ....

Christopher Maher has been admitted for day surgery to have a lesion removed from his left arm. He has nil known allergies, and is to start a course of oral penicillin for 5 days postoperatively. He has been told that he will be given the first dose in theatre.

Christine Maher is being admitted for day surgery to remove an orthopaedic pin in her left ankle. Christine needs antibiotic cover for 10 days; she is allergic to penicillin.

Using this example, write some of the potential outcomes of mixing up these two medication charts.

Locate the areas in the client identification panel that would prevent these errors from being made.

Adverse reactions and allergies

In regard to the medication chart, there are a number of specific areas that are included on the Australian NIMC, the NRMC and the New Zealand National Medication Chart. The first of these is the text box for allergies and adverse reactions (Figure 3.2).

FIGURE 3.2 Adverse reactions and allergies box (a) Allergies and adverse reactions chart (Australian) (b) NRMC allergies and adverse drug reactions

(a)

Attach ADR sticker

Allergies and adverse drug reactions (ADR)		
□ Nil known □ Unknown (tick appropriate box or complete details below)		
Medicine (or other)	Reaction / type / date	Initials

Sign .... Print .... Date ....

(b)

Allergies & Adverse Drug Reactions (ADR)	
□ Yes **DRUG ALERT LABEL** ATTACH ALERT LABEL HERE AND WHERE INDICATED INSIDE CHART □ Nil Known	
Drug (or other)	Reaction / type / date

Sign _____   Print name _____   Date ___ / ___ / ___

Prescribing officers, nurses and pharmacists are all responsible for making sure that this section is completed fully and updated where possible. This area of the medication chart needs to be filled in along with the signature of the person who is completing it. An adverse reaction sticker is also required in the boxes indicating an adverse reaction. If the client has no known allergies, then the 'nil known' or 'unknown' allergy check box needs to be filled in and the signature, printed surname and date completed sections filled at the bottom of the field.

Once only, premedication and nurse-initiated medications

In Australia, health agencies have guidelines in place that allow for nurse-initiated medication or standing orders (see Figure 3.3). The guidelines allow for a certain range of medications to be initiated by a nurse qualified to administer medication. The guidelines also nominate a range of medicine that is allowed to be administered, but they also specify a limitation on the number of times that the administration can happen. Typically, this list includes simple analgesics (such as paracetamol), aperients, antacids, cough suppressants, sublingual nitrates, inhaled bronchodilators, artificial tears, sodium chloride 0.9% flush or intravenous (IV) infusion to keep IV lines patent as directed by local policy.

This field in the medication chart needs to include:
- the date the medicine was prescribed
- the generic name of the medicine
- the route of administration
- the dose of the medicine and the date and time that it is to be given
- the prescriber's name with their printed surname (printed surname not required in NZ).

When the medicine has been given, the medication record needs to have:
- the initials of the person who has administered it
- the time it was given.

Agency policy needs to be consulted for nurse-initiated medication. The drugs and poisons legislation in Australian states and territories allows a certain range of medication to be nurse-initiated from the Schedule 2 and 3 (S2 and S3) list of medications, though this is always governed by agency policy (i.e. a medication that may be nurse-initiated at one hospital may not be permitted at a different hospital in the same area).

FIGURE 3.3 Once only, premedication and nurse-initiated medicines charts

(a) Once only and nurse initiated medicines and premedications (Australian)

(b) NRMC Nurse Initiated Medicine

Nurse Initiated Medicine				Indication / instruction	Date	Time	Dose	Inits	Date	Time	Dose	Inits
Nurse Initiated Medicine			Strength									
Date	Route	Dose	Frequency									
/ /20												
RN Signature		RN Name (Print)										

WORKED EXAMPLE 3.1

🔲 CLINICAL CASE STUDY

It is 1000 hrs on 23 August when you answer the call bell for your client, who tells you that they are constipated. You check the medication chart for the client and find that they have not had any medication for constipation ordered. You check for allergies and note that they have 'nil known allergies' written on their medication chart. You decide to nurse-initiate 20 mL lactulose. Write up the medication chart for nurse-initiated orders.

Facility/service: _Sunnyside Healthcare_

Ward/unit: _6G_

Medicine chart no. _1_ of _1_

Additional charts
☐ Iv fluid ☐ Bgl/insulin ☐ Acute pain ☐ Other
☐ Palliative care ☐ Chemotherapy ☐ Iv heparin

Once only and nurse initiated medicines and pre-medications

Date prescribed	Medicine (print generic name)	Route	Dose	Date/time of dose	Prescriber/Nurse Initiator (NI) Signature	Print your name	Given by	Time given	Pharmacy
23/08/XX	lactulose	PO	20 mL	23.08/1000 hrs	G Winkler	G Winkler	GW	1010	

Using the supplied medication chart fields, fill in the forms for the following scenarios.

1   It is 1430 hrs on 21 September. Your female client has called to tell you that her eyes feel dry and sore. She blames this on the air conditioning in the hospital. You examine her eyes and note them to be slightly red, but not inflamed. You decide to nurse-initiate some Refresh Tears® as a simple lubricant until she can be reviewed by her doctor the following day. Write this order on the self-initiated field of the medication chart.

2   It is 1745 hrs on 14 April. Your male client has been transferred to your facility from the emergency department of the local hospital. He has remembered that the nurses had commented that his IV cannula will need to be flushed every 4 hours to maintain patency. You decide to nurse-initiate 5 mL normal saline 0.9% IV. Write this on the medication chart in the supplied field.

Facility/service: ....

Ward/unit: ....

Medicine chart no. .... **of** ....

Additional charts

☐ Iv fluid ☐ Bgl/insulin ☐ Acute pain ☐ Other
☐ Palliative care ☐ Chemotherapy ☐ Iv heparin

Once only and nurse initiated medicines and pre-medications

Date prescribed	Medicine (print generic name)	Route	Dose	Date/time of dose	Prescriber/Nurse Initiator (NI) Signature Print your name	Given by	Time given	Pharmacy

Facility/service: ....

Ward/unit: ....

Medicine chart no. .... **of** ....

Additional charts

☐ Iv fluid ☐ Bgl/insulin ☐ Acute pain ☐ Other
☐ Palliative care ☐ Chemotherapy ☐ Iv heparin

Once only and nurse initiated medicines and pre-medications

Date prescribed	Medicine (print generic name)	Route	Dose	Date/time of dose	Prescriber/Nurse Initiator (NI) Signature Print your name	Given by	Time given	Pharmacy

Telephone/verbal orders

Telephone orders (Figure 3.4) must have the following fields identified inside the area designed for documenting this particular form of medication order:

- the date the medicine was prescribed
- the generic name of the medicine
- the route the medicine is to be given
- the dose of the medicine
- the date and the time the medicine is to be administered
- the name of the prescriber ordering the medicine

- the initials of the two nurses that have heard and confirmed the telephone order (this is dependent upon agency policy as some hospitals do not require two nurses to listen to the telephone order)
- the time of administration of the medicine. The New Zealand National Medication Chart also requires both of the nurses who have witnessed the telephone order to also be the same nurses who check the medication administration.

The order MUST be confirmed in writing within 24 hours – either by a signature on the medication chart beside the prescriber name or in some other format, such as digitally on an electronic medication chart, a faxed order or in writing by the prescriber.

FIGURE 3.4 Telephone orders (a) Telephone orders (Australian) (b) Telephone order (NRMC)

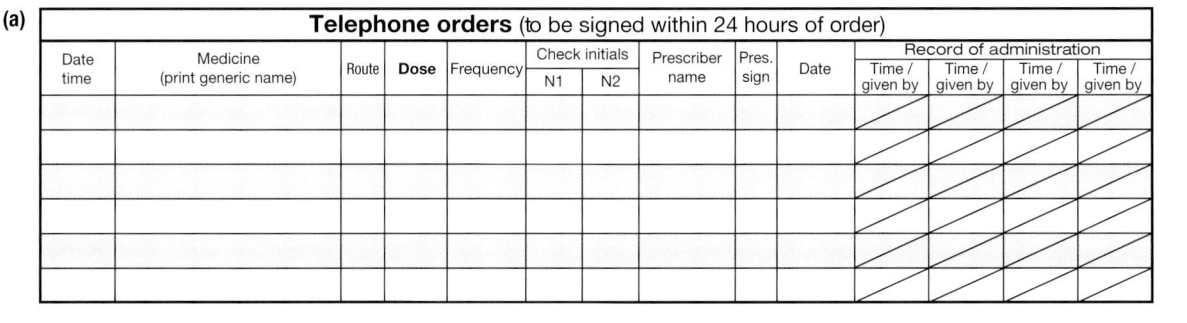

(a)

Telephone orders (to be signed within 24 hours of order)													
Date time	Medicine (print generic name)	Route	**Dose**	Frequency	Check initials		Prescriber name	Pres. sign	Date	Record of administration			
					N1	N2				Time / given by	Time / given by	Time / given by	Time / given by

(b)

Telephone Orders												
Medicine .... **Strength**	Dose	Reason ordered		Date								
	Route	Additional instructions		Time								
				Dose								
	Frequency			Initial								
	Start Date / /20	Signature 1 Date / /20		Date								
	Stop Date / /20	Signature 2 Date / /20		Time								
				Dose								
Prescriber name		Prescriber signature Date / /20		Initial								

WORKED EXAMPLE 3.2

 CLINICAL CASE STUDY

You are working in a small private hospital on an evening shift. Your 65-year-old client, who is nil orally, has fallen in the corridor of the hospital and has sustained a very nasty skin tear. You are going to dress the wounds, but need to address the severe pain that the client has before commencing the dressing.

You phone her doctor, Dr Rounds, who gives you a telephone order for 10 mg morphine IM prior to the dressing. You have asked your co-worker, Michelle Anders, to witness the telephone order. Fill in the telephone order on the medication chart.

Telephone orders (to be signed within 24 hours of order)												
Date time	Medicine (print generic name)	Route	Dose	Frequency	Check initials N1	Check initials N2	Prescriber name	Pres. sign	Date	Record of administration Time / given by	Time / given by	Time / given by	Time / given by
23/08, 1900	morphine	IM	10 mg	stat	FH	MA	Rounds		23/08/XX	1910 FH			

ACTIVITY 3.3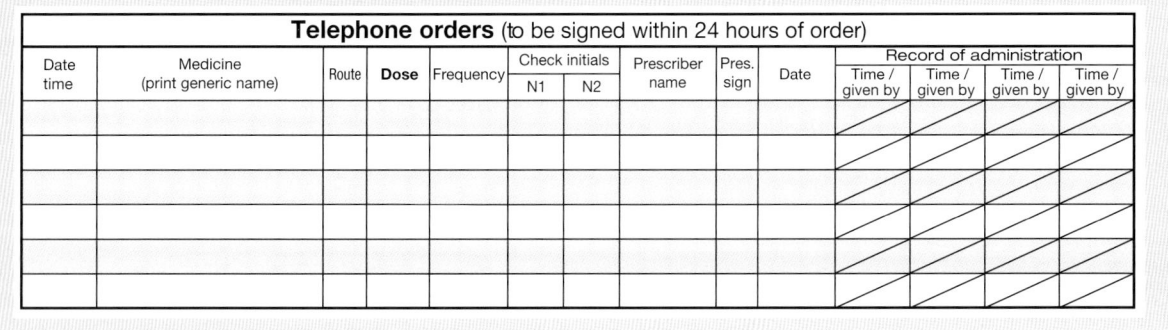

1 It is 1000 hrs on 15 October and during hourly rounding your client tells you that they have developed a reaction to some of the flowers in their room, and they have hay fever.

You remove the flowers and call their doctor, who orders fexofenadine hydrochloride 180 mg. Dr Rose tells you he will write up a daily dose when he visits in the evening. You ask your co-worker Heather Wattle to witness the order and co-sign the administration. Fill in the telephone orders for this situation.

Date time	Medicine (print generic name)	Route	**Dose**	Frequency	Check initials N1	Check initials N2	Prescriber name	Pres. sign	Date	Record of administration Time / given by	Record of administration Time / given by	Record of administration Time / given by	Record of administration Time / given by
Telephone orders (to be signed within 24 hours of order)													

Regular medications

The regular medication section of the medication chart is only a valid document if all of the sections of the chart have been filled in by the prescriber (see **Figure 3.5**).

The date field for this chart is to contain the date that the medication order was commenced for this admission. The date is not to be written as the date the medication chart was commenced or the date it has been rewritten.

The generic name of the medicine is considered to be best practice; however, it is not a legal requirement. This is to stop any medication errors from combining generic and trade names on the same chart. The only time that a medication should be written as a trade name is if the medication is a

FIGURE 3.5 Regular medications (a) Australian National Inpatient Medication Chart (b) National Residential Medication Chart (Aus)

(a) Regular medicines

Year 20	Date and month ⟶													
PRESCRIBER MUST ENTER administration times ⟶														

Date | Medicine (print generic name) | Tick if slow release
Route | Dose | Frequency and NOW enter times ⟶
Indication | | Pharmacy
Prescriber signature | Print your name | Contact

Continue on discharge? Yes / No
Dispense? Yes / No
Duration:........days Qty:..........
Date:..........

(b)

REGULAR MEDICINES 9 to 17	Date Times

Regular Medicines/Form | Strength

9

Route | Dose | Frequency and **NOW** Enter Times ⟶

Date of Prescribing | Prescriber Signature
/ /20

Not a valid prescription unless completed

☐ ☐ ☐ ☐ Streamlined authority code

☐ (✓)Brand substitution not permitted

☐ (✓) PBS ☐ (✓) RPBS ☐ (✓) CTG

Prescriber Name (Print)

Start Date
/ /20 Initial

Stop Date
☐ (✓) Tick if valid for duration of chart **OR**
Stop Date / /20 Initial

(✓) Tick appropriate box
☐ Commence Immediately ☐ Next Pack
Not a valid prescription unless completed

combined preparation of medication or if the trade name is specifically required (e.g. warfarin). In this case, it is unlikely that the hospital will stock more than one form of the medication. Examples of these types of medications are Panadol Osteo high dose (paracetamol) and Estalis continuous 50/140 (50 microg 17-β-oestradiol/140 microg norethisterone acetate).

The Australian NIMC also has a red box that needs to be ticked if the medication is to be given in a slow-release format. This is also a safety mechanism to ensure the client receives the correct form of the medication.

There is a pharmacy field at the base of each date column in the medication chart that indicates the chart has been reviewed by a pharmacist.

In regard to the NIMC, the prescriber has an opportunity to indicate that the medicine is to be continued on discharge, the duration of the order, whether it needs to be dispensed and the quantity of medicine to be dispensed. If this area has been filled by the prescriber, a side panel gives them the ability to sign the order and the pharmacist the ability to acknowlege the order.

WORKED EXAMPLE 3.3

🔍 CLINICAL CASE STUDY

It is 0800 hrs on 28 August. You are checking through the medication chart for Hannah Wines. You notice that she is due to have escitalopram 20 mg at 0800. Administer the medication using your normal checking procedures, then complete the administration record.

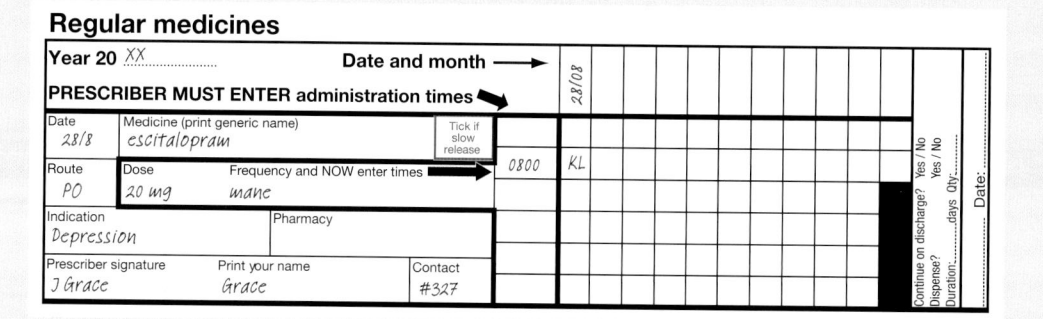

Using the supplied medication chart fields, fill in the forms for the following scenarios.

1   It is 0800 hrs on 20 August. You are checking through the medication chart for John James. You notice that he has been prescribed lamotrigine 100 mg BD (twice daily). His morning dose is now due. Administer the medication using your normal checking procedures, and then complete the administration record.

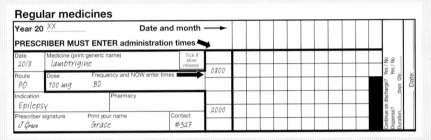

2   It is 0800 hrs on 20 August. You are checking through the medication chart for Christopher Johns. You notice that he is due to have bisoprolol 10 mg at 0800. Administer the medication using your normal checking procedures, and then complete the administration record.

Regular medicines

Year 20 XX   Date and month ⟶

PRESCRIBER MUST ENTER administration times

Date 20/8	Medicine (print generic name) bisoprolol	Tick if slow release									
Route PO	Dose 10 mg	Frequency and NOW enter times mane	0800								
Indication Hypertension		Pharmacy									
Prescriber signature J Grace	Print your name Grace	Contact #327									

PRN medications

PRN medications are medications that are prescribed to be given 'as required' to the client (Figure 3.6). The medication order needs to include:

- the date the medicine was ordered
- the generic name of the medicine
- the dose and frequency of the administration
- the route of administration

- the indication for use
- the maximum daily dose that can be given.

The health professional administering the medicine must record:

- the actual dose that has been given
- the route of administration
- the date and time of administration
- their signature.

FIGURE 3.6 PRN medications (a) Australian National Inpatient Medication Chart (b) Australian National Residential Medication Chart

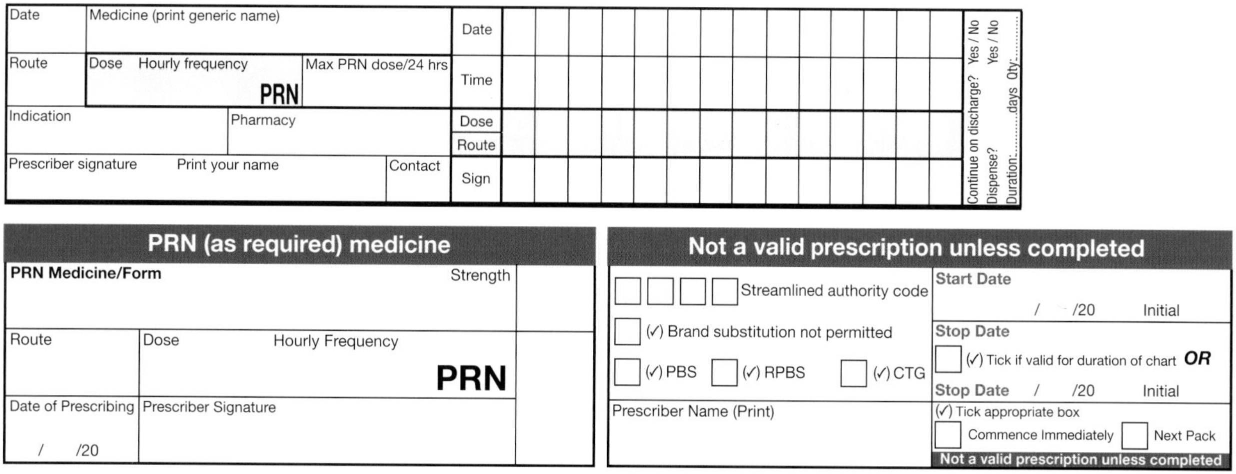

CLINICAL CASE STUDY

It is 1000 hrs on 17 August when your client tells you that they have pain. You check the medication chart for the client and find that they have a number of options for PRN medication. You check for allergies and note that they have 'nil known allergies' written on their medication chart. You decide to give them paracetamol 1 g. Write up the medication chart for the PRN orders.

Date 16/8	Medicine (print generic name) paracetamol			Date	16/8	16/8	17/8	17/8	17/8						Continue on discharge? Yes / No
Route PO	Dose 1 g	Hourly frequency 4/24 **PRN**	Max PRN dose/24 hrs 4 g	Time	1000	1600	0100	0500	1000						Dispense? Yes / No
Indication Pain		Pharmacy		Dose	1 g	1 g	1 g	1 g	1 g						Duration:.........days Qty:
				Route	PO	PO	PO	PO	PO						
Prescriber signature J Grace	Print your name Grace		Contact #321	Sign	TM	BB	EB	SB	EM						

Using the supplied medication chart fields, fill in the forms for the following scenarios.

1   It is 1100 hrs on 17 August when you check your client, who tells you that they still have pain. They are rating their pain at 6 out of 10 on the pain scale. You check the medication chart for the client and find that they have a number of options for PRN medication. You check for allergies and note that they have 'nil known allergies' written on their medication chart. You decide to give them morphine 5 mg IM. Write up the medication chart for the PRN orders.

>>

>>

Date 17/8	Medicine (print generic name) *morphine*			Date												Yes / No Yes / No Qty......
Route IM	Dose 5 mg	Hourly frequency 4/24 **PRN**	Max PRN dose/24 hrs 30 mg	Time												
Indication *Pain*		Pharmacy		Dose												Continue on discharge? Dispense? days Duration:......
				Route												
Prescriber signature *J Grace*	Print your name *Grace*		Contact #321	Sign												

2   It is 1130 hrs on 17 August when your client tells you that they are feeling nauseated, but their pain is now controlled. You check the medication chart for the client and find that they have an order for metoclopramide 10 mg IM for nausea. You check the medication chart for allergies and note that they have allergies to most anti-emetic medications except metoclopramide. You give them another IM injection – this one to control the nausea they have. Write up the medication chart for the PRN orders.

Date 17/8	Medicine (print generic name) *metoclopramide*			Date												Yes / No Yes / No Qty......
Route IM	Dose 10 mg	Hourly frequency 6/24 **PRN**	Max PRN dose/24 hrs 40 mg	Time												
Indication *Nausea*		Pharmacy		Dose												Continue on discharge? Dispense? days Duration:......
				Route												
Prescriber signature *J Grace*	Print your name *Grace*		Contact #321	Sign												

VTE prophylaxis

The purpose of the VTE prophylaxis field is to ensure that the client's risk of developing a venous thromboembolism (VTE) has been assessed (see **Figure 3.7**). If the client has been identified as requiring VTE prophylaxis, the medication required will be captured in this field and authorised by the prescriber's signature. The NIMC also allows for identification of any mechanical VTE prophylaxis to be used, allowing for nurse initiation of the

FIGURE 3.7 The VTE prophylaxis section on the NIMC (Australia)

Using the VTE prophylaxis section on the NIMC

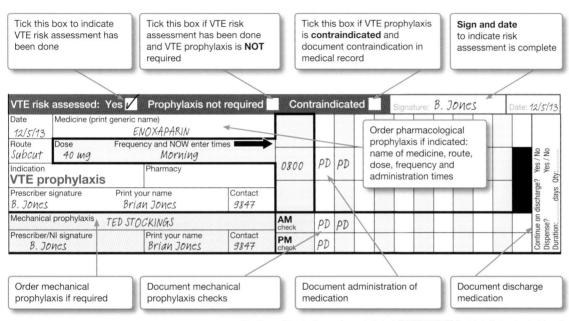

Tick this box to indicate VTE risk assessment has been done

Tick this box if VTE risk assessment has been done and VTE prophylaxis is **NOT** required

Tick this box if VTE prophylaxis is **contraindicated** and document contraindication in medical record

Sign and date to indicate risk assessment is complete

Order pharmacological prophylaxis if indicated: name of medicine, route, dose, frequency and administration times

Order mechanical prophylaxis if required

Document mechanical prophylaxis checks

Document administration of medication

Document discharge medication

https://www.safetyandquality.gov.au/wp-content/uploads/2012/02/NIMC-VTE-Prophylaxis-Poster-external-printing.pdf same if identified by hospital policy. An example of this may be the use of graduated compression stockings.

The New Zealand National Medication Chart also has a field designed to capture whether the client has been assessed for VTE risk and a summary of the VTE prophylaxis being used.

Warfarin orders

The Australian NIMC includes warfarin labelled in red (Figure 3.8). This is to highlight that the medication is a high-risk medication. The guidelines that accompany this chart recommend having a set time of 1600 hrs as an administration time. This allows time for the INR to be processed and the medication dose to be written for the following day without the need to chase results after-hours. The target INR needs to be included on the medication order, as does the indication for treating the client with warfarin.

The medication chart recommends that the INR result is recorded along with the prescriber's initials and the initials of both the administering nurse and the nurse checking the dose of warfarin.

In the acute setting, the medication chart includes a text box that records the client receiving education regarding warfarin and their own warfarin book (Figure 3.9). This is a record that can be used, if needed, to mitigate risks of prescribing and administering a dangerous drug.

For an example of an NRMC for warfarin orders see Figure 3.10(b) on page 81.

FIGURE 3.8 Warfarin orders (Australian)

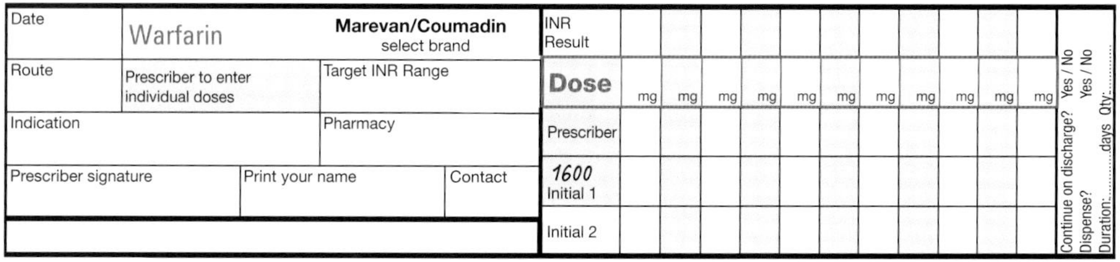

FIGURE 3.9 Warfarin education record (Australian)

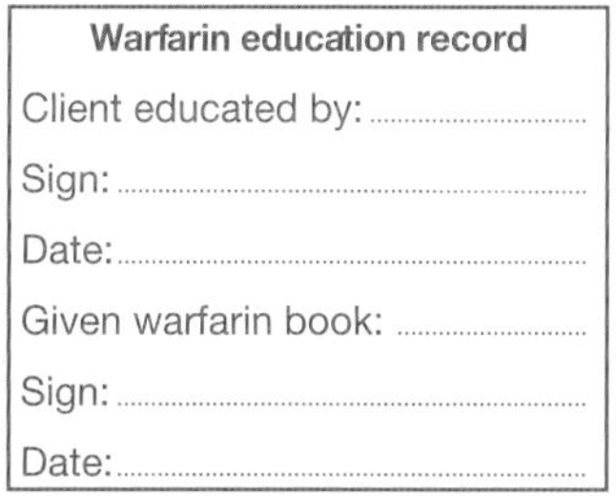

CLINICAL CASE STUDY

It is 1600 hrs on 18 August. You check the medication chart for your client who has been commenced on warfarin for atrial fibrillation. The doctor has ordered the new dose for warfarin.

You administer this dose and sign the medication record, using your initials, AB. You have the dose checked by Zara Smith.

Date 15/8	Warfarin	(Marevan/Coumadin) select brand		INR Result	1.2	1.3	1.4	1.6								Yes/No Yes/No
					15/8	16/8	17/8	18/8								
Route PO	Prescriber to enter individual doses	Target INR Range 2–3		**Dose**	2 mg	3 mg	3 mg	3 mg	mg	mg	mg	mg	mg	mg	mg	
Indication Atrial fibrillation		Pharmacy		Prescriber	JG	JG	JG	JG								Continue on discharge?
Prescriber signature J Grace	Print your name GRACE		Contact #321	**1600** Initial 1	KR	NR	FM	AB								Dispense? days Qty:
				Initial 2	VB	SM	CR	ZS								Duration:

Using the supplied medication chart fields, fill in the forms for the following scenarios.

1 It is now 1600 hrs on 19 August. You check the medication chart for your client who has been commenced on warfarin for atrial fibrillation. The prescriber has ordered the new dose for warfarin. You administer this dose and sign the medication record.

>>

Date 15/8	Warfarin	(Marevan)/Coumadin) select brand	INR Result	15/8 1.2	16/8 1.3	17/8 1.4	18/8 1.6	19/8 1.8						
Route PO	Prescriber to enter individual doses	Target INR Range 2–3	**Dose**	2 mg	3 mg	3 mg	3 mg	3 mg	mg	mg	mg	mg	mg	mg
Indication Atrial fibrillation		Pharmacy	Prescriber	JG	JG	JG	JG	JG						
Prescriber signature J Grace	Print your name GRACE	Contact #321	1600 Initial 1	KR	NR	FM	AB							
			Initial 2	VB	SM	CR	ZS							

Continue on discharge? Yes / No — Dispense? Yes / No — Duration: .... days — Qty:

2 It is 1600 hrs on 20 August. You check the medication chart for your client who is prescribed warfarin for atrial fibrillation.

The prescriber has ordered the new dose for warfarin. You administer this dose and sign the medication record.

Date 15/8	Warfarin	(Marevan)/Coumadin) select brand	INR Result	15/8 1.2	16/8 1.3	17/8 1.4	18/8 1.6	19/8 1.8	20/8 2.1					
Route PO	Prescriber to enter individual doses	Target INR Range 2–3	**Dose**	2 mg	3 mg	3 mg	3 mg	3 mg	2 mg	mg	mg	mg	mg
Indication Atrial fibrillation		Pharmacy	Prescriber	JG	JG	JG	JG	JG	JG				
Prescriber signature J Grace	Print your name GRACE	Contact #321	1600 Initial 1	KR	NR	FM	AB	RS					
			Initial 2	VB	SM	CR	ZS	BS					

Continue on discharge? Yes / No — Dispense? Yes / No — Duration: .... days — Qty:

Variable dose medication

The variable dosage medication sections on the Australian NIMC and NRMC have been included to capture the specific nature of medications such as corticosteroids, which often have a varying dosage (**Figure 3.10**). These medications are often missed if they are included on the once only section of the medication chart, and as such have now been captured in an area that allows for varying dosage. These orders need to be signed on an individual basis by the prescriber, as they are individual medication orders.

FIGURE 3.10 (a) Variable dose medication (Australian) (b) Variable dose medicine (NRMC)

(a) **Regular medicines**

Year 20	Date and month ⟶										

Variable dose medicine

Drug level

Date	Medicine (print generic name)	Time level taken

Dose

Route	Frequency	Prescriber

Prescriber to enter dose times and individual dose

Indication	Pharmacy	Time to be given: ....

Prescriber signature	Print your name	Contact	Time given

Continue on discharge? Yes / No
Dispense? Yes / No
Duration:........ days Qty:........
Date:

(b) **Variable dose medicine* (not insulin) e.g. Warfarin**

* This page to be used to prescribe different strengths of ONE medicine only

√ Box where required

P
N A
O C
N K
E
D

VARIABLE DOSE MEDICINE (Not Insulin) eg. Warfarin

Variable Dose Medicine/Form		Strength

Route	Dose	Frequency

Date of Prescribing	Prescriber Signature

Time

AM

PM

Not a valid prescription unless completed

☐ ☐ ☐ ☐ Streamlined authority code

☐ (✓) Brand substitution not permitted

☐ (✓) PBS ☐ (✓) RPBS ☐ (✓) CTG

Prescriber Name (Print)

Start Date
/   /20   Initial

Stop Date
☐ (✓) Tick if valid for duration of chart **OR**
Stop Date   /   /20   Initial

(✓) Tick appropriate box
☐ Commence Immediately   ☐ Next Pack
Not a valid prescription unless completed

Month 1	Month of		20													
Date ⟶	1	2	3	4	5	6	7	8	9	10	11	12	13	14	15	16
Pathology result																
Dose prescribed	mg	mg	mg	mg	mg	mg	mg	mg	mg	mg	mg	mg	mg	mg	mg	mg
Dose given	mg	mg	mg	mg	mg	mg	mg	mg	mg	mg	mg	mg	mg	mg	mg	mg
Time																
Initial 1																
Initial 2																

© Compact Business Systems 2013

WORKED EXAMPLE 3.6

🔍 CLINICAL CASE STUDY

It is 0800 hrs on 21 August. You check the medication chart for your client Noeline Johns, who is on a tapering dose of prednisolone for treatment of a severe exacerbation of asthma.

She has been on 45 mg daily of prednisolone and is now reducing her dosages as per the medication record. Complete the medication chart for the variable dose record.

Regular medicine

Year 20 XX			Date and month ➞	21/8	22/8	23/8									
Variable dose medicine			Drug level												
Date	Medicine (print generic name)		Time level taken												
20/8	prednisolone		**Dose**	40 mg	35 mg	30 mg						Yes / No	Yes / No	Date:	
Route	Frequency														
PO	mane		Prescriber	JG	JG	JG									
	Prescriber to enter dose times and individual dose														
Indication		Pharmacy	Time to be given:									Continue on discharge?	Dispense?	Duration:......days Qty:......	
Asthma			0800	TR											
Prescriber signature	Print your name	Contact	Time given												
J Grace	Grace	#321		0800											

ACTIVITY 3.7

Using the supplied medication chart fields, fill in the forms for the following scenarios.

1   It is the following day, 22 August, at 0800. Noeline Johns is due to receive the next dose of prednisolone. This has been ordered in the variable dosage section of her medication chart. Complete the medication chart for the variable dosage record.

Regular medicine

Year 20 XX   **Date and month** ⟶   21/8 22/8 23/8

Variable dose medicine

Date 20/8	Medicine (print generic name) prednisolone	Drug level			
		Time level taken			
Route PO	Frequency mane	**Dose**	40 mg	35 mg	30 mg
	Prescriber to enter dose times and individual dose	Prescriber	JG	JG	JG
Indication Asthma	Pharmacy	Time to be given: 0800	TR		
Prescriber signature J Grace	Print your name Grace	Contact #321	Time given	0800	

Continue on discharge? Yes / No Dispense? Yes / No Duration: ...... days Qty ...... Date: ......

---

2   It is the following day, 23 August, at 0800. Noeline Johns is due to receive the next dose of prednisolone. This has been ordered in the variable dosage section of her medication chart. Complete the medication chart for the variable dosage record.

Regular medicine

Year 20 XX   **Date and month** ⟶   21/8 22/8 23/8

Variable dose medicine

Date 20/8	Medicine (print generic name) prednisolone	Drug level			
		Time level taken			
Route PO	Frequency mane	**Dose**	40 mg	35 mg	30 mg
	Prescriber to enter dose times and individual dose	Prescriber	JG	JG	JG
Indication Asthma	Pharmacy	Time to be given: 0800	TR	TR	
Prescriber signature J Grace	Print your name Grace	Contact #321	Time given	0800	0800

Continue on discharge? Yes / No Dispense? Yes / No Duration: ...... days Qty ...... Date: ......

National Residential Medication Chart

The NRMC has additional fields designed to reduce medication errors and to ensure that the resident receives their medication as ordered, at the appropriate time (see Figure 3.11). Monitoring of an acceptable level of blood sugars and administration of insulin is captured on the same part of the medication chart to ensure that information regarding blood glucose levels (BGLs) and insulin delivery are together.

FIGURE 3.11 NRMC insulin and BGL monitoring chart

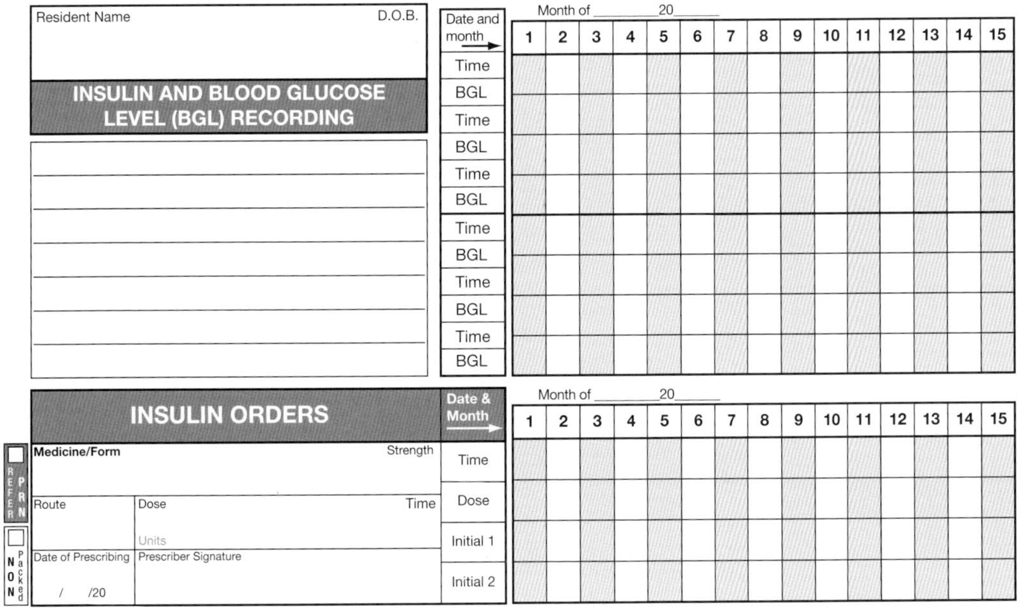

Seven 'rights' for safe medication administration

Health professionals learn the five 'rights' to medication administration early in their career. What is not covered in the five rights is the subject of many medication administration errors:

- Health professionals need to know the reason the medicine is being administered, thus the *right* reason. This helps ensure the medicine has been ordered for the right person.
- To complete medication administration, the medication chart needs to be signed – the *right* documentation.

Some examples of abnormalities with medication charts that can be checked by completing the '7 rights' and the '10 steps' (below) procedures are the following:

- Your client has been given a diagnosis of a subdural haemorrhage. You check the medication chart and find an order for digoxin 0.125 mg mane. When you check the client's medical history, you find no reference to a cardiac disease. You *need* to question this order.
- Your client is admitted for nursing care after a total knee replacement. You check their medication chart and notice an order for warfarin 2 mg. When you check the client's medical history, you find no reference to blood clots, prosthetic valves or cardiac arrhythmias. You *need* to question this order.
- Your client is admitted for antibiotic cover for a sepsis. You check their medication chart and note an order for gentamycin. When you check the client's medical history, you find they have a history of renal failure. You *need* to question this order.

SAFETY

SEVEN RIGHTS FOR SAFE MEDICATION ADMINISTRATION

1 **RIGHT** drug
2 **RIGHT** client (three identifiers)
3 **RIGHT** dose
4 **RIGHT** time
5 **RIGHT** route
6 **RIGHT** reason
7 **RIGHT** documentation

10 steps for safe use of a medication chart

The '10 steps for safe use of a medication chart' has been designed to provide you with a fail-safe method of ensuring that medication errors associated with the use of a medication chart are minimised. This guideline has been provided in all chapters to encourage familiarity with the steps and to allow you to build them into your everyday practice.

SAFETY

10 STEPS FOR SAFE USE OF A MEDICATION CHART

Step 1 Scan medication chart to ensure the prescription(s) are legal and are able to be used.

Step 2 Check which medicines are due/available to administer now.

Step 3 Check for any interactions or contraindications. If medicines have a risk of serious adverse effects, then ensure you are able to monitor/manage these safely.

Step 4 Check that the dosage and route are appropriate for the client's condition.

Step 5 Assess the client to see if the medicine(s) are suitable for them at this time. Ensure no allergies or contraindications to this medicine.

Step 6 Think about this dose – is it logical (e.g. you would not expect to give more than a couple of tablets or a few mL out of a bottle)?

Step 7 Convert all measurements to the same units and then perform dosage calculations using either the formula or the proportions method. This ensures the correct amount of medicine is given.

Step 8 Administer the medicine following the '7 rights', ensuring the client understands and consents to this.

Step 9 Sign/document the medicine as administered on the appropriate charts.

Step 10 Assess the client for any adverse effects.

4 USING QUALITY AND RISK MANAGEMENT PRINCIPLES IN DOSAGE CALCULATIONS

Introduction

Quality care is an obvious goal for all health professionals; this means striving for a degree of excellence in all their work. Dosage calculations performed incorrectly are *not* quality care and can put clients (as well as health professionals) at significant risk. Errors in dosage calculations are totally avoidable. It is therefore vital that health professionals are able to perform these calculations correctly every time.

The World Health Organization (WHO; 2023) has highlighted medication errors and unsafe practices as 'the leading cause of injury and avoidable harm in health care systems across the world', estimated to cost US$42 billion each year. In order to achieve high-quality client care, health professionals must understand the risks and be able to implement appropriate strategies to prevent or manage them. This chapter discusses the basic principles of quality and risk management and their impact on dosage calculations.

Quality in the use and administration of medicines

In 1985, the WHO developed a 'Rational Use of Medicines' agenda and encouraged the global community to develop policies to ensure medicines were being used safely.

Both Australia and New Zealand responded positively to this. Australia developed a National Medicines Policy with 'Quality use of medicines' as one of its central objectives, while New Zealand established the National Medication Safety Programme to reduce harm to clients from medication errors across the whole health and disability sector (Te Tahu Hauora Health Quality & Safety Commission, 2023). These policies have been updated for contemporary practice and guide the use and supply of medicines in both countries, with a significant focus on 'quality use of medicines'.

The term 'quality use of medicines' refers to the way that health professionals prescribe and administer medicines (including prescription and over-the-counter preparations), as well as how consumers take these medicines. Quality use of medicines includes considering whether a medicine or non-medicine option would be the best choice for a client. It also includes monitoring clients' responses to medicines so that medicines can be altered when necessary to provide the best health outcomes for the client (Australian Government Department of Health and Aged Care, 2022). Refer to the Safety box for an overview of 'quality use of medicines'.

All health professionals have an important role to play in optimising the health and safety of people using medicines. As a result of this, they should all be familiar with the aims and elements of 'quality use of medicines'; this involves government regulators, prescribers, pharmacists, consumers, pharmaceutical companies and all health professionals working with clients who use medicines.

Technically, 'quality use of medicines' and the selection/use of medicines is not directly concerned with dosage calculations. However, it is important that health professionals consider the bigger picture when administering medicines to

clients – if people do not receive the correct or appropriate dose of a medicine, then this is not 'quality use of medicines'. There are obviously inherent risks associated with errors in dosage calculations.

If dosage calculations are performed incorrectly, the client is placed at risk of harm. There are numerous risk management strategies that can be used to prevent this.

Principles of risk management

Risk to the client and health professional is very real where medicine administration is concerned. A good appreciation of these risks is warranted and health professionals should be well versed in what risks are likely/possible and how to assess, prevent and manage them.

Risk assessment and management is specifically included as part of the National Clinical Governance Standard with the Australian Commission on Safety and Quality in Health Care. It clearly states that risk management should be performed regularly as part of a continuous quality improvement framework with the aim of improving the quality of healthcare and ensuring professional standards are maintained (Australian Commission on Safety & Quality in Health Care, 2023).

Reporting of risks is vital to this quality improvement process and all health professionals should report actual and 'near miss' medication errors in order to highlight these risks. If medication errors or near misses are reported, then individual behaviours and/or systems may be adapted to prevent these recurring in the future.

It is beyond the scope of this chapter to fully discuss the principles of risk management and quality improvement frameworks; however, it is helpful for all health professionals to

SAFETY ⚠

QUALITY USE OF MEDICINES

Quality use of medicines means all health professionals need to do the following to keep clients safe:

- select management options wisely
- choose suitable medicines if a medicine is considered necessary
- administer medicines safely and effectively.

From Department of Health and Aged Care http://www.health.gov.au
\> Health products and medicines \> Medicines
\> National Medicines Policy \> Quality Use of Medicines.

know the potential risks in medication dosage calculations and what factors may have an impact on these.

Risks with dosage calculations

Factors that can influence dosage calculation errors

Numerous factors can contribute to medication calculation errors (Australian Commission on Safety and Quality in Health Care, 2023; World Health Organization, 2023). Some of the key factors that focus on the healthcare professional include:

- attitude of health professionals towards their chance of making an error (e.g. overconfidence or thinking this is 'routine')
- fear of blame or legal ramifications
- fatigue
- stress
- interruptions
- incorrect formula or incorrect use of a formula
- mathematical errors
- unclear medication order (see Figure 4.1)
- misinterpreting medication order or medicine label (see Figures 4.2 and 4.3)
- high workload
- distraction
- no logic check performed – not checking to see if the amount of medicine they have calculated seems correct (e.g. if a calculation said to give 12 tablets, this does not sound correct)
- inability to see the full picture (i.e. tunnel-vision focus)
- system errors (e.g. inadequate staffing levels)
- inexperience
- similar packaging for different medicines
- double-checking (where there is confirmation biases – where both checkers assume the other person has checked correctly, which results in neither person checking the medication/dose properly)
- single checking (where no logic check is performed or where calculation has been performed incorrectly)
  - polypharmacy (where a client is on numerous medications at the same time)
  - poor coordination of care
  - poor medication management at transitions of care (i.e. moving between one health facility and another).

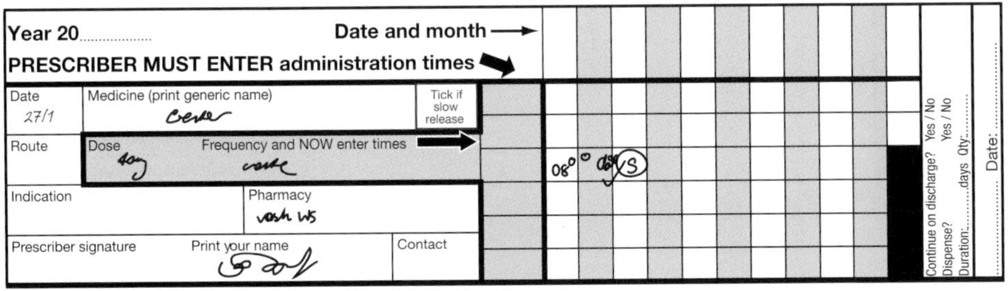

FIGURE 4.1 Unclear medication order

FIGURE 4.2 Similar medication labels – different doses of Rifadin
(a) Rifadin 300 mg (b) Rifadin 150 mg

(a)

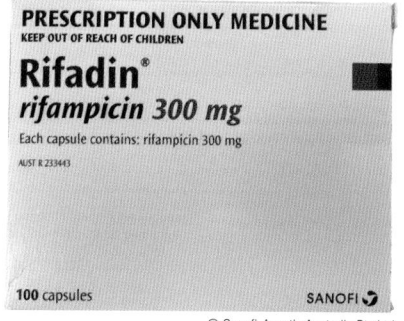

© Sanofi-Aventis Australia Pty Ltd

(b)

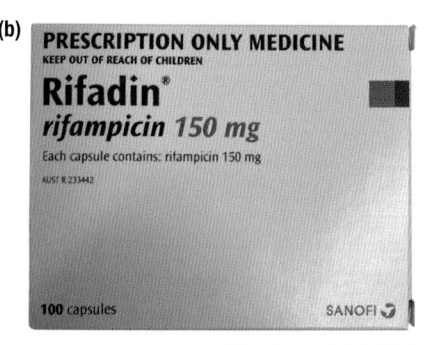

© Sanofi-Aventis Australia Pty Ltd

FIGURE 4.3 Similar medication labels – different doses of Efexor
(a) Efexor 150 mg (b) Efexor 37.5 mg

(a)

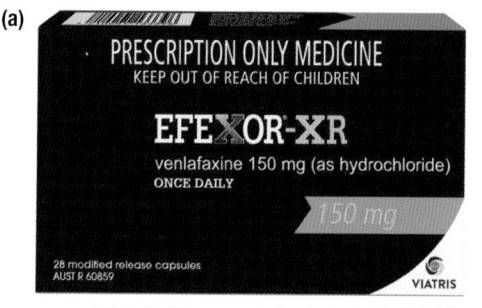

(b)

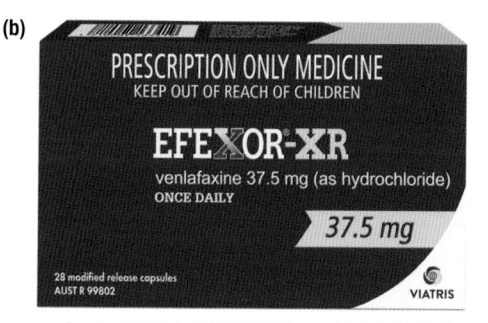

(Note that the medication packages used represent Australian packages at the specified date of publication and are reproduced for educational purposes only.)

Identifying potential dosage calculation errors

In general terms, medication errors can occur when the incorrect medication or dose is given. It could also involve the wrong route of administration or giving the medicine to the wrong client. Other medication errors involve giving the medicine at the wrong time or when the client's clinical condition would indicate the medicine is not appropriate.

Dosage calculation errors may lead to medication administration errors; it is important to note that these are different errors and the strategies for preventing dosage calculation errors are not necessarily the same as those for preventing medication administration errors.

This text does not focus on medication administration errors – there are many pharmacology/health discipline texts that cover this well. However, the next sections discuss some of the key points pertaining to dosage calculation errors and how these may be prevented.

Strategies that can help reduce the incidence of dosage calculation errors

Dosage calculation formulae are often incorrectly remembered or applied, and they can cause a great deal of stress for health professionals when trying to use them. There are numerous formulae that need to be recalled if this is the method chosen by the health professional to calculate medication doses. In the following chapters, we will illustrate the safe use of these formulae; however, we also offer an alternative to this with demonstration of how to perform the proportions method of dosage calculations. The proportions method allows health professionals to use one approach to all calculations and never have to remember and use a formula. Proficiency in a non-formula-based method of dosage calculations is one strategy against errors (Greenfield, Whelan & Cohn, 2006). Examples of this method may be seen in this chapter; however, Chapter 5 has further information on how to perform these calculations.

Some clinical agencies require health professionals to 'double-check' specific medicines or calculations before administering a medicine to a client. This is most often required as a matter of agency policy rather than a point of law. However, many agencies also require double-checking of 'drugs of dependence', intravenous (IV) preparations/infusions or other medicines. Health professionals need to be aware that double-checking can actually lead to medication errors, as the first checker may assume that any mistakes will be picked up by the second checker. Conversely, the second checker may assume that the first checker would not have made a mistake. This can lead to a 'half-check' instead of a double-check, which can increase the risk of error – be mindful of this when participating in double-checking practices. Single-checking policies also carry risk with the possibility that the health professional who does the calculation and administration independently does not have their work scrutinised for errors.

Thinking about what the expected amount of medicine should be is an important strategy in minimising calculation errors. This is often referred to as a 'logic check'. This check ensures the person performing the dosage calculation thinks about what the answer/amount of medication should be in approximate terms.

Worked example 4.1 illustrates how to perform this calculation using both the formula and the proportions methods; both of these approaches will be covered further in Chapter 5.

WORKED EXAMPLE 4.1

If a health professional has to administer 120 mg of amoxycillin, roughly how many millilitres (mL) would you expect to have to give?

If we consider that the dose is 120 mg and that the bottle contains 500 mg/5 mL, this means that in 1 mL there is 100 mg – so we need more than 1 mL. However, if we were to give 2 mL, then that would be double the amount, meaning that there is 200 mg in 2 mL and that is too much. So a logic check here would indicate that we would expect our dosage calculation to give an answer between 1 mL and 2 mL.

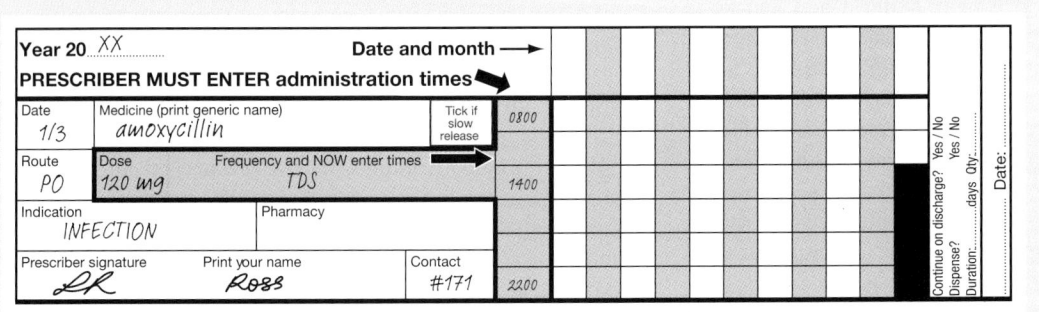

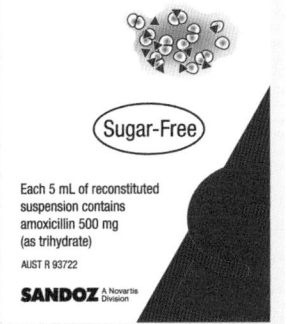

Formula method

(see Chapter 5 for more information about how to perform this type of calculation)

Let's work out the correct answer:

$$\text{Dose} = \frac{\text{strength required}}{\text{stock strength}} \times \text{volume}$$

$$\text{Dose} = \frac{120\ \text{mg}}{500\ \text{mg}} \times 5\ \text{mL}$$

Dose = 1.2 mL of amoxycillin

(120 ÷ 500 then × 5)

Proportions method

(see Chapter 5 for more information about how to perform this type of calculation)

If we have:	500 mg = 5 mL
Then we want:	120 mg = x mL

> Ensure you put the same units on the same side of the equation (i.e. here both equations have mg on the left side).

Cross-multiply: 500 mg = 5 mL
                  120 mg = x mL

> Multiply everything diagonally (i.e. 500 × x = 500x and 120 × 5 = 600)

So: $500x = 600$

Solve for x: $\dfrac{500x}{500} = \dfrac{600}{500}$

> Divide both sides by 500 to get x by itself.

x = 1.2 mL of amoxycillin

Errors concerned with dosage calculations can be approached using a three-step process as shown below.

SAFETY

THREE-STEP APPROACH TO DOSAGE CALCULATIONS

Step 1	Convert	Ensure that all measurements are in the same system of measurement and the same size unit of measurement. If not, convert before proceeding.
Step 2	Think	Estimate what is a reasonable amount of the medicine to administer.
Step 3	Calculate	Apply the formula: dose = $\dfrac{\text{strength required}}{\text{stock strength}} \times$ volume

Let's take this three-step process further in order to ensure an overall systematic process for calculating doses and establishing which medicines are due/available to give to a client. The '10 steps for safe use of a medication chart' incorporates the three-step process and ensures the health professional is checking the prescription, the client, the situation, the dosage and the follow-up care/documentation.

SAFETY

10 STEPS FOR SAFE USE OF A MEDICATION CHART

Note where the logic check is performed in Step 6.

Step 1   Scan medication chart to ensure the prescription(s) meet legal requirements and are able to be used.

Step 2   Check which medicines are due/available to administer now.

Step 3   Check for any interactions or contraindications. If medicines have a risk of serious adverse effects, then ensure you are able to monitor/manage these safely.

Step 4   Check that the dosage and route are appropriate for the client's condition.

Step 5   Assess the client to see if the medicine(s) are suitable for them at this time. Ensure no allergies or contraindications to this medicine.

Step 6   Think about this dose – is it logical (e.g. you would not expect to give more than a couple of tablets or a few mL out of a bottle)?

Step 7   Convert all measurements to the same units, then perform dosage calculations using either the formula or the proportions method. This ensures the correct amount of medicine is given.

Step 8   Administer the medicine following the '7 rights', ensuring the client understands and consents to this.

Step 9   Sign/document the medicine as administered on the appropriate charts.

Step 10   Assess the client for any adverse effects.

Refer to the prescriptions below with their corresponding medication labels. Perform a logic check for the following (i.e. estimate how much medication you expect to give).

1   Digoxin

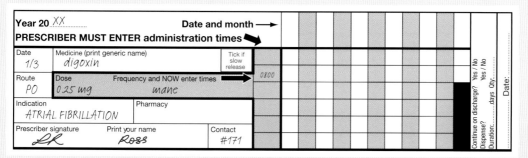

\>\>

2 Phenytoin

Year 20 XX Date and month →												
PRESCRIBER MUST ENTER administration times ↘												
Date 1/3	Medicine (print generic name) phenytoin	Tick if slow release										Continue on discharge? Yes / No
Route PO	Dose 50 mg	Frequency and NOW enter times → bd	0800									Dispense? Yes / No
Indication EPILEPSY		Pharmacy										Duration: ...... days Qty: ......
Prescriber signature LR	Print your name ROSS	Contact #171	2000									Date: ......

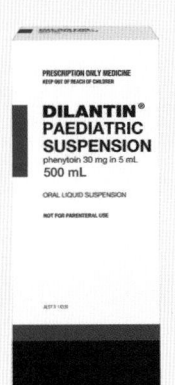

DILANTIN® is a Viatris company trade mark.
Copyright © 2022 Viatris Inc. All rights reserved.

3 Haloperidol

Date 1/3	Medicine (print generic name) haloperidol		Date											Continue on discharge? Yes / No
Route IV	Dose 3 mg Hourly frequency 4–6 hrly **PRN**	Max PRN dose/24 hrs 15 mg	Time											Dispense? Yes / No
Indication Agitation		Pharmacy	Dose											Duration: ...... days Qty: ......
			Route											
Prescriber signature LR	Print your name ROSS	Contact #171	Sign											Date: ......

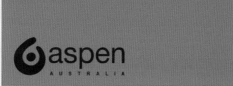

PRESCRIPTION ONLY MEDICINE
KEEP OUT OF REACH OF CHILDREN

10 Ampoules of 1 mL

Serenace Injection

5mg Haloperidol

Each 1 mL Ampoule contains:
HALOPERIDOL 5 mg
INTRAMUSCULAR OR INTRAVENOUS

Excipients: (s)-Lactic acid 0.02 mL/mL
Sodium hydroxide 1.8 mg/mL
Water for injections q.s. 1.0 mL

These ampoules should not be exposed to light

STORE BELOW 30°C.

See enclosed leaflet for directions

In Australia, Consumer Medicine Information is
available from your pharmacist or
www.aspencmi.com.au   *AUST R 188367*

aspen
AUSTRALIA

© Aspen Pharmacare

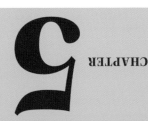

5

GENERAL DOSAGE CALCULATIONS

Introduction

In general terms, dosage calculations may be completed using two main methods – specific dosage formulae and general mathematics (often using a proportions method):

- The formulae method can be of benefit when an individual is not confident with the mathematics behind the calculation (although simple mathematical principles are always required to use the formulae correctly).

- The mathematical approach means that there is only one standard approach to all medication calculations and this removes the need for remembering complex formulae and knowing which formula to use in each situation.

There are different benefits to each method and it is up to the individual to find which method suits them best. A health professional who may struggle to remember a formula may find it easier to use the proportions method, whereas a different health professional who struggles with mathematical principles may find it easier to remember and apply a formula. However, please note that there is no formula for every circumstance, and

mathematical principles will be required to use and bridge the formulae in most circumstances.

This chapter introduces both the proportions and the formulae methods for calculation. The types of medication calculations covered in this chapter include tablets/capsules, liquids and injections.

Medication calculations: dose per kilogram

Some medicines have individualised doses based on a client's weight (for both children and adults). Therefore, sometimes health professionals need to calculate this. Usually, these are referred to as 'dose per kilo' calculations (also written as dose/kg), but may also be called weight/kg or mg/kg calculations.

Formula 4 illustrates how to calculate this, however, it can easily be done without remembering a formula, by using basic mathematics. If a client's weight is not in kilograms, their weight should first be converted to this. Chapter 7 goes into further detail on these calculations and demonstrates how these medication orders are documented on the medication chart.

FORMULA 4 – DOSE/PER KILOGRAM

Dose to be given = recommended dose (mg/kg) ×
weight (kg)

Where: 'dose/kg' has been prescribed or recommended in a medicine handbook (e.g. *Australian Medicines Handbook*).

WORKED EXAMPLE 5.1

 CLINICAL CASE STUDY

Sebastian Newell is a 7-year-old boy requiring the antibiotic Cefaclor for a chest infection. He weighs 24 kg.

When looking up the expected medication for this medicine, it says the recommended dose for this medicine is as follows:

Dosage: Cefaclor
Adult: 250–500 mg every 8 hours
Child: 15 mg/kg every 8 hours

Source: *Australian Medicines Handbook*, https://amhonline.amh.net.au/

(Note that with this particular medication, it is only the child dose that is mg/kg; the adult dose is not weight-dependent.)

What is the expected dose for Sebastian?

Dose to be given = dose (mg/kg) × weight (kg)
Dose = 15 mg/kg × 24 kg
= 360 mg Cefaclor

ACTIVITY 5.1

Calculate the expected dose for the client in the following practice questions.

1   Gentamicin is recommended at a dose of 4–7 mg/kg for adults. What dose range would you expect for a man weighing 85 kg?
2   A 13 kg child is prescribed cefotaxime. The recommended dose for this medicine is 25 mg/kg. What dose would you expect to administer to this child?
3   A 93 kg man is prescribed vancomycin at a dose of 30 mg/kg daily. What dose would you expect to administer to this man?

Medication calculations: tablets and capsules

Tablets and capsules are the most common preparations for oral medication administration. Tablets contain the medicine (plus other inactive ingredients) in a compressed form that are often 'scored', indicating where they can be broken into halves or quarters (though this is only for certain medicines, and should only be done if absolutely necessary as the accuracy of a dose may be at risk when breaking tablets into quarters).

Capsules have the medicine contained inside a gelatine covering, with the medication often in a powdered or pellet form. Capsules are not scored and cannot safely be split/broken up to give less than the full amount of the medication.

There are a number of other forms of oral medicines such as caplets and wafers, but in general the calculations are all performed exactly the same (although some of these preparations cannot be split into halves).

Some capsules and tablets can be opened or crushed into food or given via enteric feeding lines for administration, but this can be dangerous for other medicines (especially sustained-release or enteric-coated preparations). See Chapter 10 for more information on this practice.

Formula 5 illustrates how to calculate dosages for tablets, capsules and liquids; however, it can easily be done using the proportions method (without remembering a formula!). Both methods are shown in the following example. Chapter 4 covered the three-step approach to dosage calculations.

SAFETY

THREE-STEP APPROACH TO DOSAGE CALCULATIONS

Step 1	Convert	Ensure that all measurements are in the same system of measurement and the same size unit of measurement. If not, convert before proceeding.
Step 2	Think	Estimate what is a reasonable amount of the medicine to administer.
Step 3	Calculate	Calculate using the proportions method or apply the formula:

$$\text{dose} = \frac{\text{strength required}}{\text{stock strength}} \times \text{volume}$$

FORMULA 5 – DOSAGE CALCULATIONS: TABLETS AND LIQUIDS

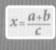

$$\text{Dose} = \frac{\text{strength required}}{\text{stock strength}} \times \text{volume}$$

You must ensure that the strength required and stock strength are both in the same units (convert to the smaller units if required).

Where:

- 'strength required' is the required dose
- 'stock strength' is the concentration of the stock you have ready to administer from
- 'volume' is the amount related to the 'stock strength' (e.g. if you have 5 mg in one tablet, the stock strength is 5 mg and the volume [quantity] is 1 tablet. If you have a liquid of concentration 10 mg/2 mL, then the stock strength is 10 mg and the volume is 2 mL).

CLINICAL CASE STUDY

Samuele Greenhill is a 9-year-old boy requiring the antihistamine cetirizine (Zyrtec) for his allergies.
The prescription is as it appears in the medication chart.
How many tablets should be given of each medicine?

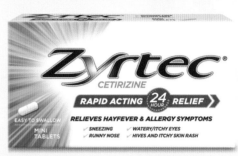

© Johnson & Johnson Pacific Pty Limited.
Each tablet of Zyrtec contains cetirizine hydrochloride 10 mg.

Regular medicines

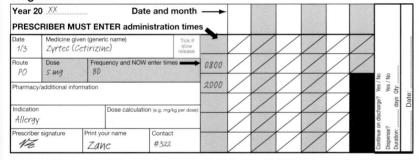

Year 20 XX	Date and month →							
PRESCRIBER MUST ENTER administration times								
Date 1/3	Medicine given (generic name) Zyrtec (Cetirizine)	Tick if slow release						
Route PO	Dose 5 mg	Frequency and NOW enter times BD →	0800					
Pharmacy/additional information			2000					
Indication Allergy	Dose calculation (e.g. mg/kg per dose):							
Prescriber signature	Print your name Zane	Contact #322						

>>

>>

Formula method

$$\text{Dose} = \frac{\text{strength required}}{\text{stock strength}} \times \text{volume}$$

$$\text{Dose} = \frac{5\,\text{mg}}{10\,\text{mg}} \times 1\,\text{tablet} \quad \boxed{(5 \div 10 \text{ then} \times 1)}$$

Dose = 0.5 or half a tablet of Zyrtec

Proportions method

| If we have: | 10 mg = 1 tablet |
| Then we want: | 5 mg = x tablets |

Cross-multiply: 10 mg = 1 tablet

5 mg = x tablets

So: $10x = 5$

Solve for x: $\dfrac{10x}{10} = \dfrac{5}{10}$

$x = 0.5$ or half a Zyrtec tablet

Ensure you put the same units on the same side of the equation (i.e. here both equations have mg on the left side).

Multiply everything diagonally (i.e. $10 \times x = 10x$ and $5 \times 1 = 5$).

Divide both sides by 10 in order to get x by itself.

ACTIVITY 5.2

Calculate how many tablets you need to administer to the client in the following practice questions.

1   Carbamazepine

Year 20 XX	Date and month →										Date:
PRESCRIBER MUST ENTER administration times →											
Date 1/3	Medicine (print generic name) *carbamazepine*	Tick if slow release									
Route PO	Dose *100 mg*	Frequency and NOW enter times *B.D.* →	0800								
Indication *EPILEPSY*	Pharmacy		2000								
Prescriber signature *VE*	Print your name *ZANE*	Contact *#322*									

PRESCRIPTION ONLY MEDICINE
KEEP OUT OF REACH OF CHILDREN

Carbamazepine Sandoz®   **200** mg

carbamazepine 200 mg
100 tablets

CG GK

Each white tablet contains carbamazepine 200 mg
AUST R 78211

SANDOZ A Novartis Division

© Sandoz Pty Ltd 2019

2 Frusemide

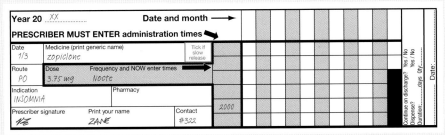

Year 20 XX	Date and month →										
PRESCRIBER MUST ENTER administration times ➤											

Date 1/3	Medicine (print generic name) frusemide		Tick if slow release	0800						Continue on discharge? Yes / No Dispense? Yes / No Duration:.....days Qty:.....	Date:
Route PO	Dose 80 mg	Frequency and NOW enter times ➤ Mane									
Indication OEDEMA		Pharmacy									
Prescriber signature VZ	Print your name ZANE		Contact #322								

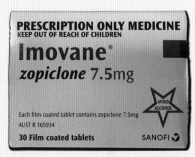

PRESCRIPTION ONLY MEDICINE
KEEP OUT OF REACH OF CHILDREN
Frusemide Sandoz® 40mg
frusemide tablets 40mg
100 tablets

100 scored white tablets
Each tablet contains 40mg frusemide.
⚖ SANDOZ AUST R 64718

DIRECTIONS FOR USE: AS PRESCRIBED BY PHYSICIAN
In Australia, the most up to date consumer medicine
information is available from your Pharmacist or from
the Sandoz website: www.sandoz.com.au
Store below 25°C. Protect from light.
Contains lactose. Gluten free. Made in India.
SANDOZ PTY LTD, ABN 60 075 449 553
54 Waterloo Road, Macquarie Park,
NSW 2113, AUSTRALIA
For further enquiries: Tel 1800 634 500 (Australia),
Tel 0800 354 335 (New Zealand)
LAB015.06

9 322838 007114

© Sandoz Pty Ltd 2019

3 Zopiclone

Year 20 XX	Date and month →										
PRESCRIBER MUST ENTER administration times ➤											

Date 1/3	Medicine (print generic name) zopiclone		Tick if slow release							Continue on discharge? Yes / No Dispense? Yes / No Duration:.....days Qty:.....	Date:
Route PO	Dose 3.75 mg	Frequency and NOW enter times ➤ Nocte		2000							
Indication INSOMNIA		Pharmacy									
Prescriber signature VZ	Print your name ZANE		Contact #322								

PRESCRIPTION ONLY MEDICINE
KEEP OUT OF REACH OF CHILDREN

Imovane®
zopiclone 7.5mg

AVOID ALCOHOL

Each film coated tablet contains zopiclone 7.5mg
AUST R 165934

30 Film coated tablets

SANOFI ✦

© Sanofi-Aventis Australia Pty Ltd

Medication calculations: liquids and concentrations

There are numerous types of liquid preparations of medicines. They have different chemical properties and disperse the medicine with the liquid in different ways. These preparations include elixirs, solutions, syrups, suspensions and mixtures. All liquid forms of medicines have a 'concentration' that is used as a basis for the calculation. Once the concentration is established, most liquid calculations are performed the same way, regardless of whether they are for oral or injectable use. The next section explains how to establish the concentration of the medicine.

Liquid concentrations and dilutions

The 'concentration' of a liquid medicine is very important to understand as it is the main information needed to complete the calculation. The concentration is a measure of the strength of the solution (i.e. a weak solution has a low concentration, whereas a strong solution has a high concentration). Concentration may be expressed in a number of ways. In general terms, it is mg/mL or units/mL that is most helpful for calculating doses; however, most topical medicines are now expressed as a percentage, which can be converted to mg/mL easily if required. Table 5.1 illustrates some of the ways the concentration of a liquid or topical cream can be expressed. Generally, it is expected that health professionals always calculate the concentration of any solution/injection that they are administering, especially in the case of those used for injection or infusion. This is a safety measure and ensures that health professionals know how much medicine is contained in 1 mL of the solution. Formula 9 on page 105 is the most commonly used formula to determine this, though a proportions approach is also easy to use.

TABLE 5.1 Concentrations of medicines

Common abbreviation	Meaning	Example
%	Proportion of the medicine out of 100.	A cream containing 3% of a medication has 3 parts medicine per 100 parts of the total volume.
% w/v	Weight of the medicine (solute) in grams divided by the total volume of the solution in millilitres (mL). Then multiplied by 100 to convert it to a percentage.	A 5% w/v solution would have 5 g of medicine (solute) dissolved in liquid to a total of 100 mL.
% v/v	Volume of the liquid medicine (solute) in millilitres divided by the total volume of the solution in millilitres. Then multiplied by 100 to convert it to a percentage.	A 1% v/v solution would have 1 mL of medicine (solute) dissolved in liquid to a total of 100 mL.
% w/w	Weight of the medicine (solute) in grams divided by the total weight of the solution in grams. Then multiplied by 100 to convert it to a percentage.	A cream containing 20 mg medicine per gram of cream. This may also be written as a 2% cream.
1 in *x* or 1:*x*	1 part of medicine/solute (could be any unit [e.g. mg, g, unit, mL]) in a total of *x* mL of liquid.	1 in 3 solution would have one part medicine combined with two parts of liquid to make a total of three parts.
mg/mL or g/mL or units/mL	The total weight (mg, g or units) that is found in 1 mL of solution.	A 20 mg/5 mL liquid would have 20 mg of medicine (solute) in 5 mL of liquid. This could also be converted to be written as 4 mg/mL.

FORMULA 6 – %w/v $x = \frac{a+b}{c}$

$$\%w/v = \frac{\text{weight of medicine}}{\text{volume of solution}} \times 100$$

FORMULA 7 – %v/v $x = \frac{a+b}{c}$

$$\%v/v = \frac{\text{volume of medicine}}{\text{volume of solution}} \times 100$$

FORMULA 8 – %w/w $x = \frac{a+b}{c}$

$$\%w/w = \frac{\text{weight of medicine}}{\text{weight of solution}} \times 100$$

FORMULA 9 $x = \frac{a+b}{c}$

$$\text{Concentration (units/mL)} = \frac{\text{amount (units)}}{\text{volume (mL)}}$$

WORKED EXAMPLE 5.3

CLINICAL CASE STUDY – PART 1

Antonio Pio is a man in the emergency department with multiple allergies.

He has the following infusions running:

- morphine 100 mg in 50 mL of normal saline
- Actrapid 100 units in 100 mL of normal saline
- heparin 25 000 units in 500 mL of normal saline.

Calculate the final concentration of these infusions in either mg/mL or units/mL.

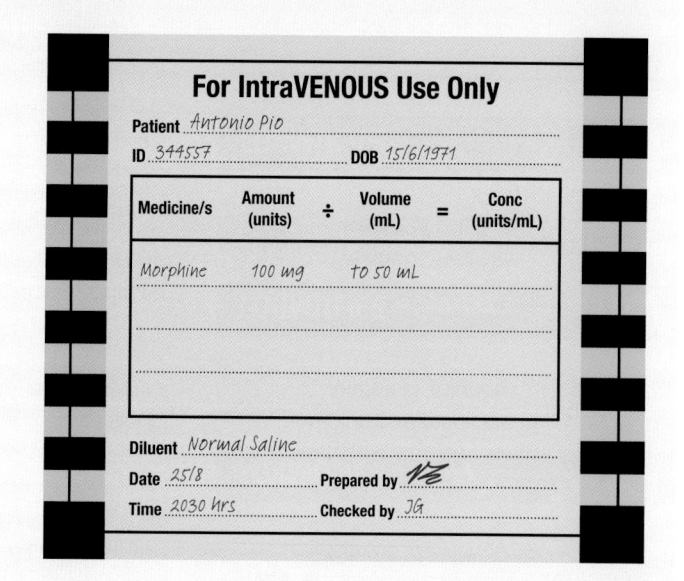

For IntraVENOUS Use Only

Patient *Antonio Pio*

ID *344557*   DOB *15/6/1971*

Medicine/s	Amount (units) ÷	Volume (mL) =	Conc (units/mL)
Morphine	*100 mg*	*to 50 mL*	

Diluent *Normal Saline*

Date *25/8*   Prepared by *VE*

Time *2030 hrs*   Checked by *JG*

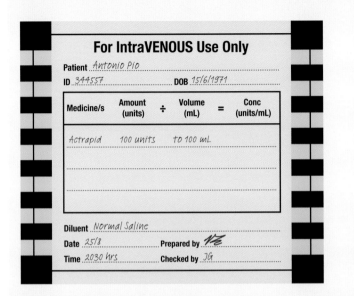

For IntraVENOUS Use Only

Patient _Antonio Pio_
ID _344557_   DOB _15/6/1971_

Medicine/s	Amount (units)	÷	Volume (mL)	=	Conc (units/mL)
Actrapid	100 units		to 100 mL		

Diluent _Normal Saline_
Date _25/8_   Prepared by _VE_
Time _2030 hrs_   Checked by _JG_

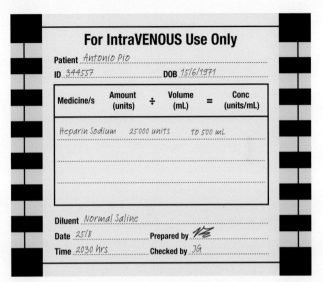

For IntraVENOUS Use Only

Patient _Antonio Pio_
ID _344557_   DOB _15/6/1971_

Medicine/s	Amount (units)	÷	Volume (mL)	=	Conc (units/mL)
Heparin Sodium	25000 units		to 500 mL		

Diluent _Normal Saline_
Date _25/8_   Prepared by _VE_
Time _2030 hrs_   Checked by _JG_

>>

MORPHINE

Formula method

Concentration (units/mL) = $\dfrac{\text{amount (units)}}{\text{volume (mL)}}$

Concentration (units/mL) = $\dfrac{100 \text{ mg}}{50 \text{ mL}}$

Concentration (units/mL) = $\dfrac{2 \text{ mg}}{\text{mL}}$

Concentration is 2 mg morphine per 1 mL of infusion.

Proportions method

If we have: 100 mg morphine = 50 mL
Then we want: x mg = 1 mL

> Ensure you keep the same units on the same side of the equation (i.e. here both equations have 'mg' on the left side).

Cross-multiply: 100 mg = 50 mL

x mg = 1 mL

> Multiply everything diagonally (i.e. $100 \times 1 = 100$ and $x \times 50 = 50x$).

So: $100 = 50x$

Solve for x: $\dfrac{100}{50} = \dfrac{50x}{50}$

> Divide both sides by 50 in order to get x by itself.

$x = 2 \text{ mg/mL}$

ACTRAPID

Formula method

$$\text{Concentration (units/mL)} = \frac{\text{amount (units)}}{\text{volume (mL)}}$$

$$\text{Concentration (units/mL)} = \frac{100 \text{ units}}{100 \text{ mL}}$$

$$\text{Concentration (units/mL)} = \frac{1 \text{ unit}}{\text{mL}}$$

Concentration is 1 unit actrapid in 1 mL of infusion.

Proportions method

If we have:	100 units Actrapid = 100 mL
Then we want:	x units = 1 mL

> Ensure you put the same units on the same side of the equation (i.e. here both equations have 'units' on the left side).

Cross-multiply:

$$100 \text{ units} = 100 \text{ mL}$$
$$x \text{ units} = 1 \text{ mL}$$

> Multiply everything diagonally (i.e. $100 \times 1 = 100$ and $x \times 100 = 100x$).

So: $100 = 100x$

Solve for x:

$$\frac{100}{100} = \frac{100x}{100}$$

> Divide both sides by 100 in order to get x by itself.

$$x = 1 \text{ unit/mL}$$

>>

>> HEPARIN

Formula method

$$\text{Concentration (units/mL)} = \frac{\text{amount (units)}}{\text{volume (mL)}}$$

$$\text{Concentration (units/mL)} = \frac{25\,000 \text{ units}}{500 \text{ mL}}$$

$$\text{Concentration (units/mL)} = \frac{50 \text{ units}}{\text{mL}}$$

Concentration is 50 units of heparin in 1 mL of infusion.

Proportions method

If we have:	25 000 units heparin = 500 mL
Then we want to know:	x units = 1 mL

> Ensure you put the same units on the same side of the equation (i.e. here both equations have 'units' on the left side).

Cross-multiply:

$$25\,000 \text{ units} = 500 \text{ mL}$$
$$x \text{ units} = 1 \text{ mL}$$

> Multiply everything diagonally
> (i.e. 25 000 × 1 = 25 000 and x × 500 = 500x).

So: $25\,000 = 500x$

Solve for x:

$$\frac{25\,000}{500} = \frac{500x}{500}$$

> Divide both sides by 500 in order to get x by itself.

$$x = 50 \text{ units/mL}$$

Antonio Pio is also prescribed the medicines found in the medication chart.

Calculate the concentration of these preparations in either mg/mL, units/mL or g/g.

Regular medicines

Year 20 XX...............	**Date and month** ⟶		
PRESCRIBER MUST ENTER administration times ➤			

Date 1/3	Medicine (print generic name) *hydrocortisone*	Tick if slow release	0800
Route *Topical*	Dose *0.5% cream*	Frequency and NOW enter times *TDS to face* ➤	
Indication *Eczema*		Pharmacy	1400
Prescriber signature ✍	Print your name *ZANE*	Contact #322	2200

Continue on discharge? Yes / No
Dispense? Yes / No
Duration:........days Qty:......
Date:......

Regular medicines

Year 20 XX...............	**Date and month** ⟶		
PRESCRIBER MUST ENTER administration times ➤			

Date 1/3	Medicine (print generic name) *timolol 0.5% eye drops*	Tick if slow release	0800
Route *Eye drops*	Dose *1 drop to both eyes*	Frequency and NOW enter times *Daily* ➤	
Indication *Glaucoma*		Pharmacy	
Prescriber signature ✍	Print your name *ZANE*	Contact #322	

Continue on discharge? Yes / No
Dispense? Yes / No
Duration:........days Qty:......
Date:......

>>

>>

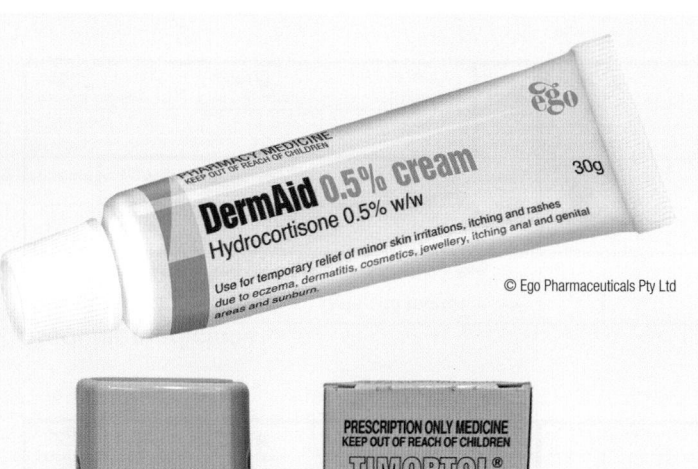

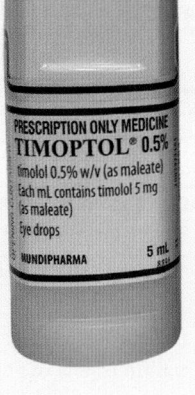

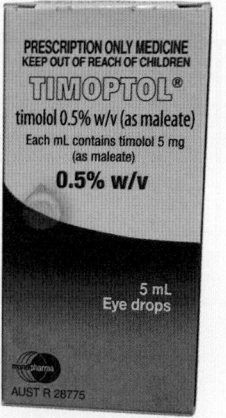

© Ego Pharmaceuticals Pty Ltd

® TIMOPTOL is a trade mark of
MUNDIPHARMA

Hydrocortisone 0.5% w/w cream

↳ 0.5% indicates 0.5 parts
hydrocortisone to
99.5% other components (cream)

↳ $\text{w/w} = \dfrac{\text{grams of medicine}}{\text{grams of total cream}}$

↳ $\dfrac{0.5\,\text{g}}{100\,\text{g}}$ $(0.5 \div 100)$

= 0.005 g/g

↳ Multiply by 1000 to convert to mg/g

0.005 × 1000 = 5 mg/g

Timolol 0.5% w/v eye drops

↳ 0.5% indicates 0.5 parts
timolol to
99.5% other components (liquid)

↳ w/v = grams per mL

↳ $\dfrac{0.5\,\text{g}}{100\,\text{mL}}$ $(0.5 \div 100)$

= 0.005 g/mL

↳ Multiply by 1000 to convert to mg/mL

0.005 × 1000 = 5 mg/mL

ACTIVITY 5.3

Calculate the concentration in the following practice questions.

1 A client is ordered a 0.05% w/w betamethasone cream. How many milligrams (mg) are in this 100 g tube?
2 A client is ordered a 1 litre 5% dextrose infusion. How many grams of dextrose are in this 1000 mL bag of fluid?
3 A client has an infusion containing 6 mg of adrenaline in 90 mL of normal saline solution. How many mg/mL is this?

Liquid dosage calculations

Liquid dosage calculations are illustrated using Formula 5; however, liquid dosage calculations can also easily be done using the proportions method (without remembering a formula!). Both methods are shown in Worked example 5.4.

WORKED EXAMPLE 5.4

 CLINICAL CASE STUDY

Stefano Napoleon is a 1-year-old boy who fell at home, breaking his arm. He has been prescribed oral paracetamol and midazolam.

The two prescriptions appear in the medication charts. What dose of each is needed?

>>

>>

PARACETAMOL

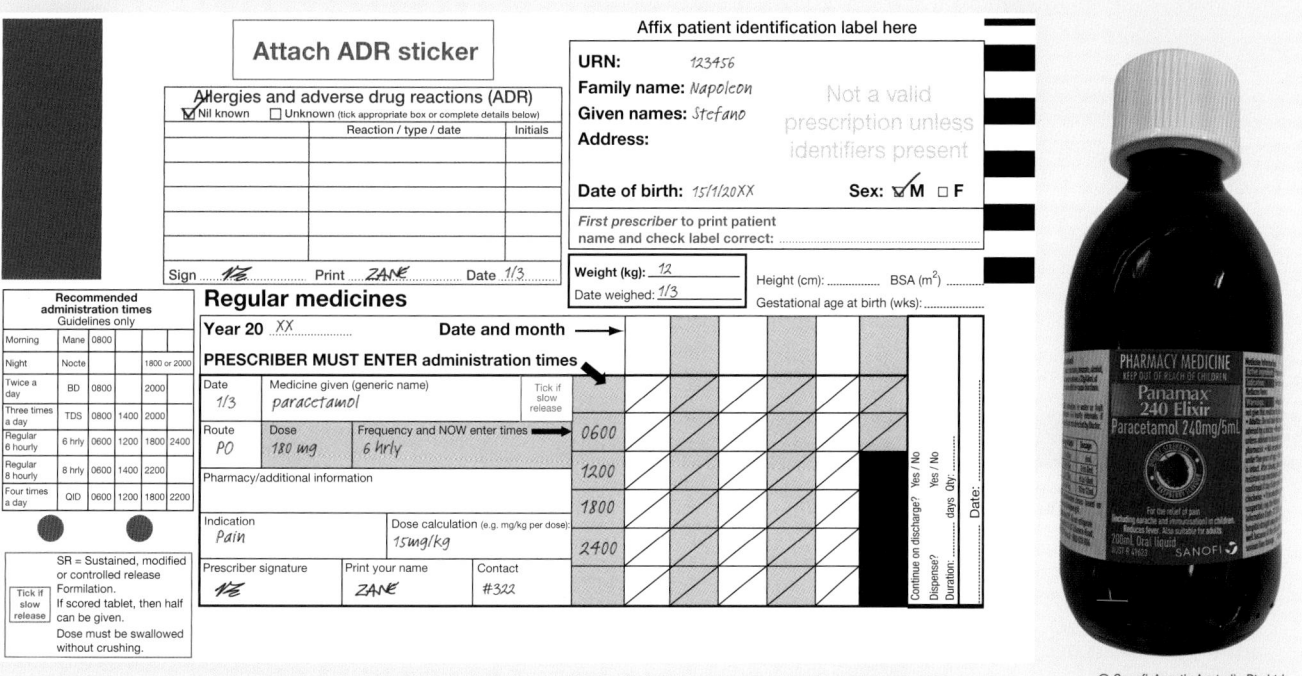

Attach ADR sticker

Allergies and adverse drug reactions (ADR)

☑ Nil known ☐ Unknown (tick appropriate box or complete details below)

	Reaction / type / date	Initials

Sign *VE* Print ZANE Date .1/3.

Affix patient identification label here

URN: 123456

Family name: Napoleon

Given names: Stefano

Address:

Not a valid prescription unless identifiers present

Date of birth: 15/1/20XX   **Sex:** ☑ M ☐ F

First prescriber to print patient name and check label correct: ....

Weight (kg): 12   Height (cm): .... BSA (m²) ....

Date weighed: 1/3   Gestational age at birth (wks): ....

Recommended administration times Guidelines only		
Morning	Mane	0800
Night	Nocte	1800 or 2000
Twice a day	BD	0800	2000
Three times a day	TDS	0800 1400 2000
Regular 6 hourly	6 hrly	0600 1200 1800 2400
Regular 8 hourly	8 hrly	0600 1400 2200
Four times a day	QID	0600 1200 1800 2200

Tick if slow release

SR = Sustained, modified or controlled release Formilation. If scored tablet, then half can be given. Dose must be swallowed without crushing.

Regular medicines

Year 20 XX ....   Date and month ⟶

PRESCRIBER MUST ENTER administration times

Date 1/3	Medicine given (generic name) *paracetamol*		Tick if slow release							
Route PO	Dose 180 mg	Frequency and NOW enter times ⟶ 6 hrly		0600						
Pharmacy/additional information				1200						
Indication Pain	Dose calculation (e.g. mg/kg per dose): 15mg/kg			1800						
Prescriber signature *VE*	Print your name ZANE	Contact #322		2400						

Continue on discharge? Yes / No
Dispense? Yes / No
Duration: .... days Qty: .... Date:

© Sanofi-Aventis Australia Pty Ltd

Formula method

$$\text{Dose} = \frac{\text{strength required}}{\text{stock strength}} \times \text{volume}$$

$$\text{Dose} = \frac{180 \text{ mg}}{240 \text{ mg}} \times 5 \text{ mL} \quad \boxed{(180 \div 240 \text{ then} \times 5)}$$

Dose = 3.75 mL paracetamol

Proportions method

If we have: 240 mg = 5 mL
Then we want: 180 mg = x mL

Ensure you put the same units on the same side of the equation (i.e. here both equations have mg on the left side).	

Cross-multiply: 240 mg = 5 mL

                    180 mg = x mL

Multiply everything diagonally (i.e. 240 $\times$ x = 240x and 180 $\times$ 5 = 900).	

So: $240x = 900$

Solve for x: $\dfrac{240x}{240} = \dfrac{900}{240}$

Divide both sides by 240 in order to get x by itself.	

                    x = 3.75 mL paracetamol

>>

>>

MIDAZOLAM

Affix patient identification label here

URN:	123456
Family name:	Napoleon
Given names:	Stefano
Address:	

Not a valid
Prescription unless
Identifiers present

Date of birth: 15.1.20XX   Sex: ☑ M ☐ F

First prescriber to print patient name
and check label correct: ....

Attach ADR sticker

See front page for details

As required
PRN
medicines

Weight (kg): ....12....
Date weighed: ...1/3....   Ward/unit:.....................

Date 1/3	Medicine (print generic name) midazolam			Date												Continue on discharge? Yes / No	Date:
Route PO	**Dose** 6 mg	Hourly frequency Stat **PRN**	Max PRN dose/24 hrs	Time												Dispense? Yes / No	
Pharmacy/additional information				**Dose**												Duration: ...... days Qty:	
Indication Anxiety pre theatre	Dose calculation (eg. mg/kg per dose) 0.5 mg/kg			Route													
Prescriber signature 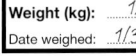	Print your name ZANE	Contact/pager # 322		Sign													

PRESCRIPTION ONLY MEDICINE
KEEP OUT OF REACH OF CHILDREN

Midazolam HCl Syrup
2 mg/mL*

*Each mL contains 2 mg midazolam (as the hydrochloride)
Orange flavour

118mL

Formula method

$$\text{Dose} = \frac{\text{strength required}}{\text{stock strength}} \times \text{volume}$$

$$\text{Dose} = \frac{6\,\text{mg}}{2\,\text{mg}} \times 1\,\text{mL} \qquad \boxed{(6 \div 2 \text{ then} \times 1)}$$

$$\text{Dose} = 3\,\text{mL}$$

So 3 mL of midazolam can be given.

Proportions method

| If we have: | 2 mg = 1 mL |
| Then we want: | 6 mg = x mL |

> Ensure you put the same units on the same side of the equation (i.e. here both equations have mg on the left side).

Cross-multiply: 2 mg = 1 mL

6 mg = x mL

> Multiply everything diagonally (i.e. $2 \times x = 2x$ $6 \times 1 = 6$).

So: $2x = 6$

Solve for x: $\dfrac{2x}{2} = \dfrac{6}{2}$

> Divide both sides by 2 in order to get x by itself.

$$x = 1.2\,\text{mL}$$

So 3 mL of midazolam can be given.

ACTIVITY 5.4

Calculate how many millilitres (mL) you need to administer to the client in the following practice questions.

1   Amoxycillin

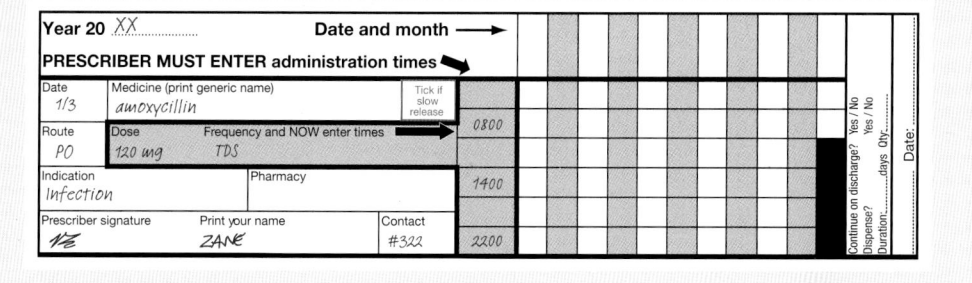

Year 20 XX	Date and month ⟶											
PRESCRIBER MUST ENTER administration times												

Date 1/3	Medicine (print generic name) amoxycillin		Tick if slow release	0800								Continue on discharge? Yes / No
Route PO	Dose 120 mg	Frequency and NOW enter times TDS										Dispense? Yes / No ......days Qty.......
Indication Infection		Pharmacy		1400								Date:
Prescriber signature *VE*	Print your name ZANE		Contact #322	2200								

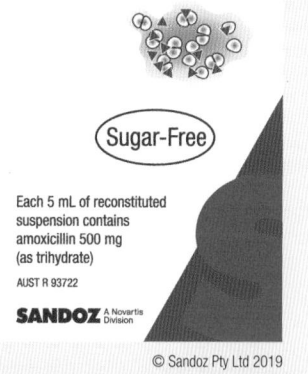

PRESCRIPTION ONLY MEDICINE
KEEP OUT OF REACH OF CHILDREN

Maxamox®

amoxicillin trihydrate 500 mg/5 mL

powder for oral suspension
100 mL (when mixed)

1 bottle

(Sugar-Free)

Each 5 mL of reconstituted
suspension contains
amoxicillin 500 mg
(as trihydrate)
AUST R 93722

SANDOZ A Novartis Division

© Sandoz Pty Ltd 2019

2 Gentamicin

Date	Medicine (print generic name)		Tick if slow release										

Year 20 XX ....   **Date and month** ➜

PRESCRIBER MUST ENTER administration times ➜

Date 1/3	Medicine (print generic name) gentamicin		Tick if slow release	0800									
Route IV	Dose 240 mg	Frequency and NOW enter times Daily ➜											
Indication Infection		Pharmacy											
Prescriber signature NE	Print your name ZANE	Contact #322											

Continue on discharge? Yes / No Dispense? Yes / No Duration:........days Qty:........ Date:

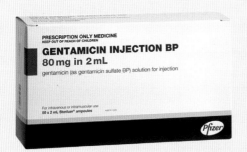

PRESCRIPTION ONLY MEDICINE
KEEP OUT OF REACH OF CHILDREN
GENTAMICIN INJECTION BP
80 mg in 2 mL
gentamicin (as gentamicin sulfate BP) solution for injection

For intravenous or intramuscular use
50 x 2 mL Steriluer® ampoules

Pfizer

© Pfizer

>>

3   Amiodarone

Facility/service:	Medicine chart no. .... of ....

Additional charts
☐ Iv fluid   ☐ Bgl/insulin   ☐ Acute pain   ☐ Other
Ward/unit: ....   ☐ Palliative care   ☐ Chemotherapy   ☐ Iv heparin

Once only and nurse initiated medicines and pre-medications

Date prescribed	Medicine (print generic name)	Route	Dose	Date/time of dose	Prescriber/Nurse Initiator (NI) Signature	Print your name	Given by	Time given	Pharmacy
1/3	amiodarone	IV	325 mg	STAT	Ƶ	ZANE			

PRESCRIPTION ONLY MEDICINE
KEEP OUT OF REACH OF CHILDREN

Cordarone X®Intravenous

amiodarone hydrochloride **150 mg/3 mL**

Sterile Amiodarone Concentrate Solution for Injection for infusion

For intravenous use

Each ampoule contains
Amiodarone hydrochloride   150 mg
Benzyl alcohol   60 mg
Polysorbate 80   300 mg
Water for injections   qs 3 mL

AUST R 15360

6 x 3 mL Ampoules   **SANOFI** 🜂

© Sanofi-Aventis Australia Pty Ltd

CHAPTER

6 INFUSION CALCULATIONS

Introduction

'Infusion' in clinical terms refers to a solution (usually of medicines, electrolytes or blood products) that is administered to a client commonly (but not always) via an intravenous route. Infusions may contain potent or toxic medicines/electrolytes and are usually regulated in terms of how fast they are administered to the client; it is for this reason that rate calculations need to be performed. To err on the side of caution, the health professional should check the medication chart and the IV infusion chart to see if the client has been prescribed a medicine to be given as part of an infusion or as a bolus dose. Careful scrutiny of these charts will allow for planning of the appropriate medicines ordered for the day.

This chapter introduces both the proportions and the formulae methods for infusion rate calculation. The chapter also describes the more common types of infusion delivery devices (gravity fed, volumetric/syringe/PCA) and appropriate calculations for these. Insulin infusion pumps are used in highly specialised areas and require more complex basal metabolic rate calculations. Since these insulin pumps are mostly set up and adjusted by clients and specialised health professionals (i.e. endocrinologists and diabetes educators), these are not covered in this chapter.

Types of infusion delivery

There are numerous types of infusion delivery devices used in healthcare. These often work on the same principles – rate in 'drops per minute' (dpm) for the gravity fed devices and rate in 'millilitres per hour' (mL/h) for the majority of pumps.

SAFETY

TIP FOR STUDENTS

All of these infusion devices must be handled with aseptic technique (for any tubing to be connected to the client). They must be properly primed with fluid before attaching to a client and starting them running, as otherwise the fluid will push a volume of air into the client, which may have serious health effects.

Infusions via gravity feed (IV drip)

Intravenous fluids or infusions that are not connected to an electronic pump to regulate flow are referred to as 'gravity feed' systems or 'IV drips'. These may be set up in a variety of ways but usually they have the intravenous solution in a flask (plastic or glass) that is attached to an administration/giving set via a sharp spike that allows the fluid to flow from the flask into the administration/giving set. There may be a burette attached between the administration/giving set and flask, depending upon the client requirements and clinical agency policy.

The gravity feed intravenous line is regulated by use of a manual roller clamp, which adjusts the diameter of the tubing in the administration/giving set and this either slows down or speeds up the rate of fluid flow (measured in drops per minute). Figure 6.1 illustrates how a gravity feed infusion is set up.

FIGURE 6.1 Gravity feed infusion (IV drip)

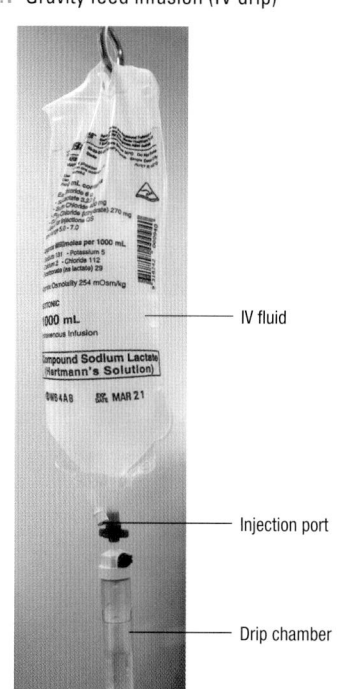

IV fluid

Injection port

Drip chamber

Kate Rafferty

TIP FOR STUDENTS

Administration/giving sets usually come with one of two drip chambers (see Figure 6.2):

- Standard (or macrodrip) giving set delivers 20 drops in each mL of fluid.
- Microdrip giving set delivers 60 drops in each mL of fluid.

FIGURE 6.2 Drip chambers for delivering IV drops

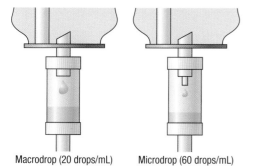

Macrodrop (20 drops/mL)   Microdrop (60 drops/mL)

Infusion (volumetric) pumps

There are many types of volumetric pumps but they mostly all set their rates in millilitres per hour (mL/h). An intravenous (IV) infusion is prepared in a flask (or sometimes in a burette or syringe) and connected to an administration/giving set (specific to the type of volumetric pump being used), which is then connected to the client's IV cannula (often a peripheral IV cannula) or access device (often a central catheter inserted into the neck, groin or subclavicular area).

The administration/giving set is inserted into the pump, which electronically regulates how much fluid can pass from the flask into the client, based on the rate set on the pump. Figure 6.3 illustrates an infusion pump.

Syringe pumps (syringe drivers)

Standard syringe pumps electronically regulate the flow of infusion that is contained in a syringe inserted into the pump. Smaller volume infusions may be prepared in appropriate-sized syringes (often 50 or 60 mL), which are attached (usually via a Luer lock) to an administration/giving set that attaches to a cannula or access device in the client.

Similar to the volumetric pump, the syringe pump electronically regulates how much fluid can pass from the syringe into the client, based on the rate that has been set. Figure 6.4 illustrates a working syringe pump.

Patient-controlled analgesia (PCA) pumps

Sometimes specialised volumetric pumps may be used to deliver analgesic infusions (e.g. narcotics) where the client requests a dose by pressing a button. These pumps allow clients a degree of freedom and choice over how much analgesia they wish to

FIGURE 6.3 Infusion pump

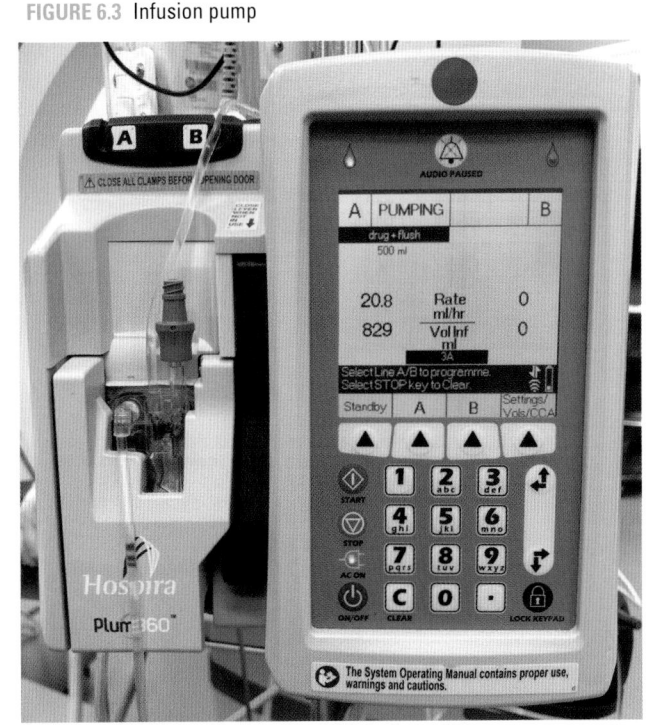

Kate Rafferty

FIGURE 6.4 Syringe pump

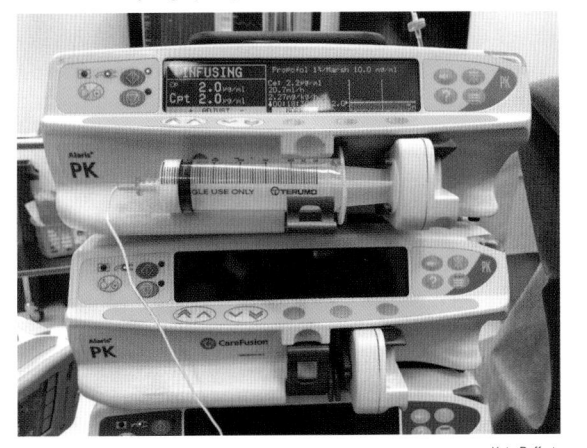

Kate Rafferty

have. PCA pumps can also be set to run a background infusion in the same way that a standard volumetric pump operates. Figure 6.5 shows a PCA pump being used.

The health professional (usually medical or nursing staff) programs the prescribed rate and volume to be administered into the pump. As part of this, a 'bolus dose' is programmed, which is the volume of infusion to be administered when a client pushes the button. There will also be a 'lockout' period set, which is the minimum time that must pass between two bolus doses. This is a safeguard against a client continually pushing the button and so accidentally overdosing on the drug in the infusion.

Similar again to volumetric pumps, the PCA pump electronically regulates how much fluid can pass from the syringe/flask into the client, based on the rate that has been set.

FIGURE 6.5 Patient-controlled analgesia (PCA) pump

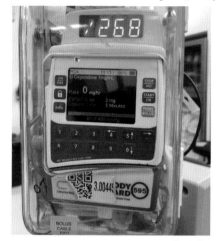

Kate Rafferty

Approaching infusion calculations

In previous chapters, we have discussed the '10 steps for safe use of a medication chart' that helps to ensure the health professional is checking the prescription, the client, the situation, the dosage and the follow-up care/documentation. It is important to think of intravenous fluids in this same way and so these 10 steps can be amended for use with infusions.

10 STEPS FOR SAFE CALCULATION OF INFUSIONS

Step 1   Scan medication chart to ensure the fluid prescription(s) are legal and are able to be used.

Step 2   Check which fluids/infusions are due to administer now.

Step 3   Check for any interactions or contraindications. All intravenous fluids have a risk of serious adverse effects (e.g. electrolyte imbalance/fluid overload). Ensure you are able to monitor/manage these safely.

Step 4   Check that the type of fluid, rate and route are appropriate for the client's condition. Think about this fluid – is it logical (e.g. you would not expect to give a client with a high sodium level a large infusion of 0.9% sodium chloride)?

Step 5   Determine how you are going to administer this fluid (e.g. via gravity feed or electronic pump). Refer to prescriber instructions, clinical agency policy, available equipment, etc.

Step 6   Calculate the rate of infusion in the appropriate format for the infusion delivery device (e.g. drops per minute [dpm] or mL/h).

Step 7   Explain to the client what you are doing and obtain verbal consent.

Step 8   Administer the fluid following the '7 rights' and clinical agency policy (e.g. timing strips or additive labels may be required). Correct aseptic technique must be used when handling all infusions and vascular access devices/cannulae.

Step 9   Sign/document the fluid order as administered on the appropriate charts (fluid prescription order and fluid balance chart, if appropriate).

Step 10   Assess the client for any adverse effects.

Calculating rates for infusions

The type of calculation required depends upon the method to be used to deliver the infusion (e.g. gravity feed infusions require the calculation of a 'drip rate' in drops per minute; volumetric/ syringe pumps require the calculation of a rate in mL/h).

For all calculations, you need to know the volume to be infused (VTBI) so that you can either set the volumetric pump or calculate the drops per minute. This is simply the amount of fluid (in millilitres) that needs to be administered to the client.

SAFETY

TIP FOR LEARNERS
When setting the volume to be infused, remember that you may have used some fluid in priming the administration/giving set, meaning a 1000 mL flask may now only contain 980 mL of fluid (or less), so always watch your infusions and stop them before the fluid runs out. Some practitioners set their volumetric pumps to 980 mL for a 1000 mL flask just to be sure that the fluid does not all run through and allow air to enter the line.

Calculating drip rate in drops per minute (dpm)

Drops per minute is the calculation used for gravity feed devices that are regulated with a manually operated roller clamp. The health professional adjusts the roller clamp and watches the number of drops that fall into the drip chamber. They count the number of drops per minute (in a similar way to counting a pulse) and adjust the roller clamp so they have the correct rate based on the number of drops that fall into the drip chamber in one full minute.

SAFETY

TIP FOR LEARNERS
When calculating drops per minute, you need to round up or down to the nearest whole number!

In order to calculate the rate of infusion in drops per minute, Formula 10 may be used.

FORMULA 10 – DROPS PER MINUTE (WHEN TIME IS KNOWN IN MINUTES)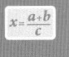

$$\text{Rate (dpm)} = \frac{\text{total volume of fluid to be infused (mL)} \times \text{number of drops per mL}}{\text{time (minutes)}}$$

Where:
   'number of drops per mL' refers to the use of either a standard giving set (macrodrip), which delivers 20 drops per mL, or a microdrip giving set, which delivers 60 drops per mL.

FORMULA 11 – DROPS PER MINUTE (WHEN TIME IS KNOWN IN HOURS)

$$\text{Rate (dpm)} = \frac{\text{total volume of fluid to be infused (mL)} \times \text{number of drops per mL}}{\text{time (hours)} \times 60}$$

WORKED EXAMPLE 6.1

 CLINICAL CASE STUDY (DROPS PER MINUTE)

Sasha Tezza is a woman requiring intravenous fluids for dehydration. She is ordered the intravenous fluids shown on the medication chart. *Assume the use of a standard giving set, which delivers 20 drops per mL.*

INTRAVENOUS FLUID TREATMENT		Sasha Tezza 27 White St Hiliary; D.O.B. 3/5/1989		BIRTHDATE	

DATE	START TIME	BOT. NO.	VOLUME	TYPE OF FLUID	ADDITIVES	RATE	DOCTOR'S SIGNATURE/ NAME	SIGNATURES 1 NURSE 2 CHECKER
27/5/XX	Stat	1	1 litre	0.9% normal saline	NIL	4 hourly	JC Connor	

>>

>>

a What is the rate of infusion (drops per minute) for this infusion?

b Sign the above drug chart appropriately as if you had commenced the infusion.

Formula method

1000 mL over 4 hours − convert to minutes:
$$4 \text{ h} \times 60 \text{ min} = 240 \text{ minutes}$$

$$\text{Rate (dpm)} = \frac{\text{total volume of fluid to be infused (mL)} \times \text{number of drops per mL}}{\text{time (minutes)}}$$

$$\text{Rate (dpm)} = \frac{1000 \text{ mL} \times 20 \text{ drops per mL}}{240 \text{ min}}$$

[macrodrip giving set delivers 20 drops per mL]

$$\text{Rate (dpm)} = \frac{20000}{240}$$

$$\text{Rate (dpm)} = 83.3333 \text{ drops per minute}$$

Round this down to 83 drops per minute.

Proportions method

If a giving set gives 20 drops per mL and we need to give a total of 1000 mL, then 20 drops/mL × 1000 = 20 000 drops in total.

If we have:	20000 drops = 240 min
Then we want:	x drops = 1 min

Ensure you put the same units on same side of the equation (i.e. both equations have drops on the left side).

Cross-multiply:
$$20000 = 240$$
$$x = 1$$

Multiply everything diagonally (i.e. 20 000 × 1 = 20 000 and 240 × x = 240x).

So: $20000 = 240x$

Solve for x:
$$\frac{20000}{240} = \frac{240x}{240}$$

Divide both sides by 240 in order to get x by itself.

$$x = 83.3333 \text{ drops per minute}$$

Round this down to 83 drops/min.

There are quick-reference tables available for looking up drops per minute rates for standard drip chambers (Table 6.1). These tables are easy to use but require the health professional to remember the drops per minute instead of being able to calculate it. If you choose to use these tables, ensure you also know how to calculate this for when non-standard volumes or times are prescribed.

TABLE 6.1 Drops per minute (dpm) expected for a 1000 mL (1 litre) flask according to the time required and the type of drip chamber giving set used

Drip chamber	Give over 1 h (60 mins)	Give over 2 h (120 mins)	Give over 4 h (240 mins)	Give over 6 h (360 mins)	Give over 8 h (480 mins)	Give over 10 h (600 mins)	Give over 12 h (720 mins)	Give over 24 h (1440 mins)
20 drops/mL	333 dpm	167 dpm	83 dpm	56 dpm	42 dpm	33 dpm	28 dpm	14 dpm
60 drops/mL	1000 dpm	500 dpm	250 dpm	167 dpm	125 dpm	100 dpm	83 dpm	42 dpm

ACTIVITY 6.1

Calculate the rate of infusion in drops per minute for the following clients.

5% GLUCOSE

1   Assume the use of a standard (macrodrip) drip chamber giving set.

INTRAVENOUS FLUID TREATMENT

DATE	START TIME	BOT. NO.	VOLUME	TYPE OF FLUID	ADDITIVES	RATE	DOCTOR'S SIGNATURE/ NAME	SIGNATURES 1 NURSE 2 CHECKER
27/5/XX	Stat	1	500 mL	5% glucose	NIL	Over 6 hours	JC Connor	

>>

>>

HARTMANNS

2 Assume the use of a standard (macrodrip) drip chamber giving set.

**INTRAVENOUS
FLUID TREATMENT**

DATE	START TIME	BOT. NO.	VOLUME	TYPE OF FLUID	ADDITIVES	RATE	DOCTOR'S SIGNATURE/ NAME	SIGNATURES 1 NURSE 2 CHECKER
27/5/XX	Stat	1	1 litre	Hartmanns	NIL	Over 12 hours	JC Connor	

0.9% NORMAL SALINE

3 Assume the use of a microdrip drip chamber giving set.

**INTRAVENOUS
FLUID TREATMENT**

DATE	START TIME	BOT. NO.	VOLUME	TYPE OF FLUID	ADDITIVES	RATE	DOCTOR'S SIGNATURE/ NAME	SIGNATURES 1 NURSE 2 CHECKER
27/5/XX	Stat	1	100 mL	0.9% normal saline	NIL	4 hourly	JC Connor	

Calculating rate of infusion in millilitres per hour (mL/h) when time is known in hours

It is useful to know how much fluid a client is receiving each hour for both documentation of fluid intake (e.g. a fluid balance chart) and also for setting electronic infusion pumps. Most volumetric/syringe pumps require the input of two variables – the volume to be infused (e.g. the amount in millilitres) and the rate of infusion (in millilitres per hour).

In order to calculate the rate of infusion in millilitres per hour, Formula 12 can be used.

An alternative way to calculate these is the proportions method (refer to Worked example 6.2).

WORKED EXAMPLE 6.2

 CLINICAL CASE STUDY (mL/h WITH TIME IN HOURS)

Basil Lucia is a man admitted to hospital requiring intravenous fluids while fasting for an operation.

He is ordered the intravenous fluids shown on the chart.

	INTRAVENOUS FLUID TREATMENT		Basil Lucia; 33 Amy Dve Seaview; D.O.B. 3/7/1990					

DATE	START TIME	BOT. NO.	VOLUME	TYPE OF FLUID	ADDITIVES	RATE	DOCTOR'S SIGNATURE/ NAME	SIGNATURES 1 NURSE 2 CHECKER
27/5/XX	Stat	1	1 litre	Hartmanns	NIL	12 hourly	JC Connor	

>>

>>

You need to use a volumetric infusion pump, which requires you to set both the volume to be infused and the rate (mL/h).
a What is the volume to be infused?
b What is the rate of infusion (mL/h) for this infusion?

a The volume to be infused is 1000 mL so this should be entered into the pump (or you may choose to enter a smaller number so the pump will alarm before the fluid runs out).

b Rate of infusion:

Formula method

Rate = mL/h

or

$$\text{Rate} = \frac{\text{total volume of fluid to be infused (mL)}}{\text{time (h)}}$$

$$\text{Rate} = \frac{1000 \text{ mL}}{12 \text{ hours}}$$

Rate = 1000 ÷ 12

Rate = 83.3333 mL/h (round down to 83 mL/h)

Proportions method

If we have: 1000 mL = over 12 hours
Then we
want: x mL = over 1 hour

> Ensure you put the same units on the same side of the equation (i.e. here both equations have mL on the left side).

Cross-multiply: 1000 mL = 12 hours

x mL = 1 h

> Multiply everything diagonally
> (i.e. 1000 × 1 = 1000 and 12 × x = 12x).

So: 1000 = 12x

Solve for x: $\dfrac{1000}{12} = \dfrac{12x}{12}$

x = 83.3333 mL/h

> Divide both sides by 12 in order to get x by itself.
>
> Round this down to 83 mL; the pump needs to be set at 83 mL/h.

Calculate the following for each question below:

a   Volume to be infused in millilitres (mL)

b   Rate of infusion (mL/h)

1   5% GLUCOSE

INTRAVENOUS FLUID TREATMENT

DATE	START TIME	BOT. NO.	VOLUME	TYPE OF FLUID	ADDITIVES	RATE	DOCTOR'S SIGNATURE/ NAME	SIGNATURES 1 NURSE 2 CHECKER
27/5/XX	Stat	1	500 mL	5% glucose	NIL	6 hourly	JC Connor	

>>

2 0.9% NORMAL SALINE

INTRAVENOUS
FLUID TREATMENT

DATE	START TIME	BOT. NO.	VOLUME	TYPE OF FLUID	ADDITIVES	RATE	DOCTOR'S SIGNATURE/ NAME	SIGNATURES 1 NURSE 2 CHECKER
27/5/XX	Stat	1	100 mL	0.9% normal saline	NIL	2 hourly	JC Connor	

3 HARTMANNS

INTRAVENOUS
FLUID TREATMENT

DATE	START TIME	BOT. NO.	VOLUME	TYPE OF FLUID	ADDITIVES	RATE	DOCTOR'S SIGNATURE/ NAME	SIGNATURES 1 NURSE 2 CHECKER
27/5/XX	Stat	1	1000 mL	Hartmanns	NIL	12 hourly	JC Connor	

Calculating rate of infusion in millilitres per hour (mL/h) when time is known in minutes

Sometimes a small amount of fluid must be administered over less than one hour and so the time is given in minutes. The calculation is basically the same as Formula 12, except the time is written in minutes and the top line of the formula is changed to account for this (see Formula 13).

WORKED EXAMPLE 6.3

 CLINICAL CASE STUDY (mL/h WITH TIME IN MINUTES)

Liliana Tosca is a 21-year-old woman requiring 60 mL of a medicine over 45 minutes for pneumonia.

You need to use a volumetric infusion pump, which requires you to set both the volume to be infused and the rate (mL/h).

a What is the volume to be infused?

b What is the rate of infusion (mL/h) for this infusion?

a The volume to be infused is 60 mL so this should be entered into the pump (or you may choose to enter a smaller number so the pump will alarm before the fluid runs out).

b Rate of infusion:

Formula method

Rate = mL/h

or

$$\text{Rate (mL/h)} = \frac{\text{total volume of fluid (mL)} \times 60}{\text{time (minutes)}}$$

$$\text{Rate (mL/h)} = \frac{60 \text{ mL} \times 60}{45 \text{ min}}$$

Rate (mL/h) = $60 \times 60 \div 45$

Rate (mL/h) = 80 mL/h

Proportions method

If we have: 60 mL = over 45 min
Then we x mL = over 60 min
want:

> Ensure you put the same units on the same side of the equation (i.e. here both equations have mL on the left side).

Cross-   60 mL = 45 min
multiply: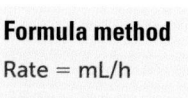
              x mL = 60 min

> Multiply everything diagonally
> (i.e. $60 \times 60 = 3600$ and $45 \times x = 45x$).

So: 3600 = 45x

Solve for x: $\dfrac{3600}{45} = \dfrac{45x}{45x}$

> Divide both sides by 45 in order to get x by itself.

              x = 80 mL/h

So the pump needs to be set at 80 mL/h.

ACTIVITY 6.3

Calculate the following practice questions.

1   A client requires 20 mL of an antibiotic over 10 minutes using a volumetric pump. Calculate the following:
   a   Volume to be infused in millilitres (mL)
   b   Rate of infusion (mL/h)
2   A child requires 10 mL of fluid over 30 minutes using a syringe pump. Calculate the following:
   a   Volume to be infused in millilitres (mL)
   b   Rate of infusion (mL/h)
3   A man is prescribed 100 mL of an intravenous medicine to be administered over 20 minutes using a volumetric pump. Calculate the following:
   a   Volume to be infused in millilitres (mL)
   b   Rate of infusion (mL/h)

Changing from a gravity feed (dpm) to a volumetric pump (mL/h)

Sometimes a client may begin an infusion on a gravity feed system (IV drip) using rate in drops per minute and then change to a volumetric pump (rate in mL/h) when one becomes available. The system may also be reversed, with a client starting an infusion using a volumetric pump and then being changed to a gravity feed (IV drip) requiring rate in drops per minute.

Once again, the rate calculation for this is mostly the same as already explained; however, the one thing that changes is the volume to be infused, since the infusion has already delivered some of the fluid in the flask (see Formula 14).

FORMULA 14 – CALCULATING 'NEW VOLUME TO BE INFUSED' (VTBI) FOR EXISTING INFUSIONS

$$x = \frac{a+b}{c}$$

New volume to be infused (mL) = total fluid (mL) – what has already been administered

WORKED EXAMPLE 6.4

 CLINICAL CASE STUDY (CHANGING FROM DROPS PER MINUTE TO mL/h)

Colorectal surgeon Adrian Doyle has prescribed intravenous fluids for his client following bowel surgery. The client currently has a 1000 mL 0.9% sodium chloride flask that started an hour ago. It is running at a 4-hourly rate (83 drops per minute) using a standard macrodrip giving set. A volumetric pump is now available.

Calculate the following:
a   What is the new rate of infusion (mL/h)?
b   What is the new volume to be infused (VTBI) in millilitres (mL)?

a   Calculate the rate as shown in previous sections – in this case, we need the rate in mL/h. (If the rate was needed in drops per minute a different formula would be used.)

$$\text{Rate} = \frac{\text{mL}}{\text{h}}$$

$$\text{Rate} = \frac{1000 \, \text{mL}}{4 \, \text{hours}}$$

$$\text{Rate} = 1000 \div 4$$

$$\text{Rate} = 250 \, \text{mL/h}$$

>>

b Since this flask has already been running for the past hour at 250 mL per hour (via a gravity feed), we assume that 250 mL has already been administered, so the remaining volume to be infused would be:

New volume to be infused

= total fluid − what has already been administered

= 1000 − 250 mL

= 750 mL

The new volume to be infused is 750 mL so this should be entered into the pump (or you may choose to enter a smaller number so the pump will alarm before the fluid runs out).

ACTIVITY 6.4

Calculate the following practice questions.

1 A client has a 1 litre IV drip running at 14 drops per minute (24-hourly rate) using a standard macrodrip giving set. It commenced 5 hours ago. A volumetric pump is now available. Calculate the following:

a New rate of infusion (mL/h)

b New volume to be infused in millilitres (mL)

2 A client has a 1 litre IV drip running at 42 drops per minute (8-hourly rate) using a standard macrodrip giving set. It commenced 3 hours ago. A volumetric pump is now available. Calculate the following:

a New rate of infusion (mL/h)

b New volume to be infused in millilitres (mL)

3 A client needs to continue their 1000 mL infusion that has been running at 83 mL/h (12-hourly rate) on a volumetric pump for the past hour. What is the rate (in drops per minute) if this were to be changed to a gravity feed system (IV drip)? Assume the use of a standard macrodrip giving set. Calculate the following:

a Rate of infusion (drops per minute)

b New volume to be infused in millilitres (mL)

How long until the infusion is finished

If an infusion is new (or even if it has already been started), it is useful to know how long until it is expected to finish (i.e. to know when to stop the infusion or change the flask). To do this, you can use Formula 15, or you could use mathematics to work it out without a formula.

WORKED EXAMPLE 6.5

 CLINICAL CASE STUDY (HOW LONG UNTIL INFUSION FINISHES)

Rupert Marta is ordered 1000 mL of 4% glucose and 0.18% sodium chloride intravenous solution. It is running at 150 mL/h and has been running for two hours.

Calculate how long until this infusion finishes.

To do this *mathematically* you could simply add up the volume already administered:

1st hour (150 mL) + 2nd hour (150 mL) = 300 mL

Then work out what you have left:

1000 mL total − 300 mL = 700 mL left

Then work out how long 700 mL would last, running at 150 mL/h:

$$\frac{700\,\text{mL}}{150\,\text{mL/h}}$$

= 700 mL ÷ 150 mL/h

= 4.66 hours left

Round this to 4.7 hours.

To do this *using the formula*:

Use Formula 14 or general mathematics to establish how much has already been administered. Since this flask has already been running for the past 2 hours at 150 mL per hour, we calculate the remaining volume to be infused to be:

New volume to be infused

= total fluid − what has already been administered

= 1000 − (150 mL + 150 mL)

= 700 mL

>>

>>

Time until finished (hours) = total fluid to be administered from now

$$= \frac{(mL)}{rate\ (mL/h)}$$

$$= \frac{700\,mL}{150\,mL/h}$$

$$= 700 \div 150$$

$$= 4.66\ hours$$

Round this to 4.7 hours.

ACTIVITY 6.5

Calculate how long it will take for the following infusions to finish.

1　A client is ordered 1000 mL of Hartmanns solution. It is running at a 4-hourly rate and was started 2 hours ago. How long until this infusion finishes?

2　A client is ordered 500 mL of a blood product. It is running at 100 mL per hour and was started 1 hour ago. How long until this infusion finishes?

3　A client is ordered 1000 mL of intravenous solution. It is running at a 10-hourly rate (using a standard macrodrip giving set) and was started 1.5 hours ago. How long until this infusion finishes?

Changes to the infusion rate

Sometimes infusions that are already running need to be sped up or slowed down. The rate calculation for this is mostly the same as already explained; however, one thing that will change is the volume to be infused, since the infusion has already delivered some of the fluid in the flask.

ACTIVITY 6.6

Calculate the following practice questions.

1　A client has a 1000 mL intravenous drip (gravity feed) running at an 8-hourly rate for the past hour. The prescriber now requires this to be sped up to a 4-hourly rate. What is the new rate in drops per minute? Assume the use of a standard macrodrip giving set.

2　At 0830 hrs, a prescriber orders the 500 mL 5% glucose infusion to be slowed down from 100 mL/h to 50 mL/h via volumetric pump. It has already been running for 30 minutes. Calculate the following:

　a　New volume to be infused in millilitres (mL)
　b　New rate (mL/h) to be set on the pump
　c　The time this infusion will end

3　A 1000 mL flask of 0.9% sodium chloride solution is to be slowed down from a 6-hourly rate to an 8-hourly rate. The infusion has only just started one minute ago. What is the new rate in drops per minute? Assume the use of a standard macrodrip giving set.

Calculating more complex rates for infusions

Chapter 9 details the calculation of more complex infusions, such as those requiring microg/min or microg/kg/min, as well as how to run a bolus dose of an infusion over a set period of time. While these types of calculations are often found in critical care and high dependency type clinical areas, it is important that all health professionals (involved with infusion management) are aware of how to perform these.

ACTIVITY 6.7

Calculate the following practice questions.

1   Your client has been ordered 1 g vancomycin, which you have reconstituted as per the instructions on page 142. Once you have drawn up the vancomycin in the required amount of water for injection, dilute this to a strength of 10 mg/mL in a burette (using saline as the diluent).

   Using the information from the *Australian Injectable Drugs Handbook*, read the information about the reconstitution and administration of vancomycin.

   a   How many millilitres of normal saline do you need to add to make this concentration?

   b   The rate of administration should not exceed 10 mg/min. What rate do you need to run this infusion to give 1 g of vancomycin?

2   Your client is ordered fentanyl at 20 microg per hour in an infusion pump. 100 microg fentanyl is diluted with normal saline 0.9% to a volume of 10 mL.

   a   Calculate the volume of medicine delivered by infusion per hour.

   b   Calculate the volume (in mL) delivered by infusion per day and the total amount of fentanyl delivered per day.

>>

VANCOMYCIN

BRAND NAME	VANCOMYCIN ALPHAPHARM, DBL, JUNO, VIATRIS
DRUG CLASS	Glycopeptide antibiotic
AVAILABILITY	Vial contains 500 mg or 1 g of vancomycin as vancomycin hydrochloride.[1]
	May also contain hydrochloric acid and/or sodium hydroxide. DBL brand also contains disodium edetate.[1]

WARNING

> Extravasation may cause tissue necrosis.[1,2]
>
> Vancomycin can cause severe infusion reactions including profound hypotension and vancomycin flushing (red man) syndrome. Do not infuse faster than the recommended rate.[1] Check your local guidelines.

pH	2.5–4.5[1]
PREPARATION	Reconstitute the 500 mg vial with 10 mL of water for injections and the 1 g vial with 20 mL of water for injections to make a concentration of 50 mg/mL.[1]
	The solution is clear and colourless to light pink or brown.[1]
	Dilute the dose to 5 mg/mL with a compatible fluid, i.e. dilute 1 g to at least 200 mL.[1]
	If necessary for fluid-restricted patients, the maximum concentration is 10 mg/mL, i.e. dilute 1 g in 100 mL.[1]
	For intravitreal injection: must be reconstituted and diluted under aseptic conditions, preferably by pharmacy.
STABILITY	Vial: store below 25 °C. Protect from light.[1]
	Reconstituted solution: stable for 24 hours at 2 to 8 °C.[1]
	Infusion solution: stable for 24 hours below 25 °C and at 2 to 8 °C.[1,2]
	For CoPAT use: infusion solutions are stable for 24 hours at up to 37 °C.[3-5]
	Infusion solutions prepared in a sterile production unit are stable for 72 hours at 37 °C or for more than 7 days at 2 to 8 °C.[2,3]

ADMINISTRATION

IM injection	Contraindicated, causes ulceration and necrosis.[1]
SUBCUT injection	Contraindicated, causes ulceration and necrosis.[1]
IV injection	Not recommended. See SPECIAL NOTES
IV infusion	See PREPARATION

> Infuse at a maximum rate of 10 mg/minute, i.e. infuse a 1 g dose over 100 minutes.[1] Use an infusion pump. See WARNING.

If necessary a 1 g dose may be infused over 1 hour. For doses over 1 g, increase the infusion time by 30 minutes for each additional 500 mg, i.e. 1.5 g over 1.5 hours and 2 g over 2 hours.[6,7]

Check your local guidelines or ask your pharmacy service for advice before proceeding. This faster rate of infusion may increase the risk of infusion reactions including severe hypotension and vancomycin flushing (red man) syndrome. Monitor blood pressure and slow the infusion if necessary. See SPECIAL NOTES.

May also be given as a continuous infusion over 24 hours.[1,8]

IV use for infants and children	Dilute to 5 mg/mL or less and infuse over at least 60 minutes. Maximum rate for doses over 500 mg is 10 mg/minute. If fluid restricted, a maximum concentration of 10 mg/mL can be infused into a central line over at least 60 minutes.[9,10]
Other	There is limited information about continuous infusions.[9,10] Seek specialist advice.
	Suitable for intravitreal injection by an ophthalmologist. Very low doses are used and special preparation is required.[11]
	Suitable for intraperitoneal administration.[12]

564 Australian Injectable Drugs Handbook 9th Edition

COMPATIBILITY

Fluids

Y-site Sodium chloride 0.9%[1], glucose 5%[2], glucose 10%[2], Hartmann's[1,2], Plasma-Lyte 148 via Y-site[13]

Y-site Aciclovir[2], amiostine[2], amiodarone[2], anidulafungin[2], aztreonam[14], buprenorphine[14], calcium chloride[1], calcium gluconate[14], caspofungin[2], cefuroxime[14], ciclosporin[14], clindamycin[14], dexamethasone[1], digoxin[14], ephedrine sulfate[14], erythromycin[14], esmolol[14], fentanyl[14], filgrastim[2], fluconazole[2], gentamicin[14], granisetron[2], hydromorphone[2], insulin (Novorapid)[15], isavuconazole[2], labetalol[2], lidocaine[14], linezolid[2], magnesium sulfate[2], metoclopramide[14], midazolam[2], morphine sulfate[2], mycophenolate mofetil[2], nicardipine[2], palonosetron[2], paracetamol[2], pethidine[2], posaconazole[1], remifentanil[2], tigecycline[2], tobramycin[14], zidovudine[2]

INCOMPATIBILITY

Fluids No information

Drugs Albumin[2], aminophylline[17], azathioprine[17], bivalirudin[2], calcium folinate[17], daptomycin[17], defibrotide[2], epoetin alfa[17], fluoxacillin[17], foscarnet[17], furosemide[17], ganciclovir[17], ketorolac[17], methylprednisolone sodium succinate[17], moxifloxacin[17], omeprazole[2], rocuronium[2], sodium bicarbonate[1], sodium valproate[17], urokinase[17]

Vancomycin is incompatible with many beta-lactam antibiotics, i.e. penicillins, cephalosporins and carbapenems.[1] Precipitation is more likely at higher concentrations of vancomycin.[2,17] Flush the line well. Ask your pharmacy service for more information.

Concentrations of vancomycin up to 5 mg/mL in sodium chloride 0.9% are compatible with piperacillin-tazobactam up to 90 mg/mL (of piperacillin) in sodium chloride 0.9%. Higher concentrations are incompatible.[16]

SPECIAL NOTES

Therapeutic monitoring may be required. Refer to your local guidelines or *Therapeutic Guidelines: Antibiotics* for recommendations.

May cause pain at the injection site and thrombophlebitis. If possible use concentrations of 2.5–5 mg/mL and rotate the infusion site.[1]

Vancomycin flushing (red man) syndrome is a histamine-mediated reaction that presents as tingling, flushing or rash of the face, neck and upper body, muscle spasm of the chest and back, and in severe cases, hypotension and shock-like symptoms. A maximum rate of infusion of 10 mg/minute is recommended. If symptoms occur, slow the rate of the infusion.[1]

Administer with caution to patients with a history of hypersensitivity to teicoplanin as cross sensitivity may occur.[1]

The injection is given orally to treat staphylococcal enterocolitis and antibiotic-associated pseudomembranous colitis produced by *Clostridium difficile*. Dilute the contents of one 500 mg vial with 30 mL of distilled water. A flavouring agent may be added to mask the offensive taste.[1]

REFERENCES

1. Product information. Available from www.tga.gov.au. Accessed 10/01/2023.
2. ASHP Injectable drug information 2021. Bethesda, MD: American Society of Health-System Pharmacists; 2021.
3. Raverby V, Ampe E, Hecq J-D, Yukens PM. Stability and compatibility of vancomycin for administration by continuous infusion. J Antimicrob Chemother 2013; 68: 1179-82.
4. Allen Jr LV. Stability of vancomycin hydrochloride in medication cassette. Int J Pharm Compd 1997; 1: 123-4.
5. Siles ML, Allen Jr LV, Prince SJ. Stability of various antibiotics kept in an insulated pouch during administration via portable infusion pump. Am J Health-Syst Pharm 1995; 52: 70-4.
6. Rybak M, Lomaestro B, Rotschafer JC, Moellering Jr R, Craig W, Billeter M, et al. Therapeutic monitoring of vancomycin in adult patients: a consensus review of the American Society of Health-System Pharmacists, the Infectious Diseases Society of America, and the Society of Infectious Diseases Pharmacists. Am J Health-Syst Pharm 2009; 66: 82-98.
7. Matsumoto K, Takesue Y, Ohmagari N, Mochizuki T, Mikamo H, Seki M, et al. Practice guidelines of therapeutic drug monitoring of vancomycin: a consensus review of the Japanese Society of Chemotherapy and the Japanese Society of Therapeutic Drug Monitoring. J Infect Chemother 2013; 19: 365-80.
8. Principles of vancomycin use (August 2020). In: Therapeutic Guidelines [internet]. Melbourne: Therapeutic Guidelines Limited; August 2022.
9. Phelps SJ, Hagemann TM, Lee KR, Thomson AU. Pediatric injectable drugs. The teddy bear book. 11th ed. Bethesda, MD: American Society of Health-System Pharmacists; 2018.
10. Paediatric Formulary Committee. BNF for children. London: BMJ group and Pharmaceutical Press; 2022-2023.
11. Endophthalmitis [April 2019]. In: Therapeutic Guidelines [internet]. Melbourne: Therapeutic Guidelines Limited; August 2022.
12. Peritonitis complicating peritoneal dialysis [April 2019]. In: Therapeutic Guidelines [internet]. Melbourne: Therapeutic Guidelines Limited; August 2022.
13. Medical information. Plasma-Lyte 148 compatibility summary. Toongabbie, NSW: Baxter; March 2022.
14. Trissel LA, Leissing NC. Trissel's Tables of physical compatibility. Lake Forest, IL: Multimatrix; 1996.
15. Voirol P, Berger-Gryllaki M, Pannatier A, Eggimann P, Sadeghipour F. Visual compatibility of insulin aspart with intravenous drugs frequently used in ICU. Eur J Hosp Pharm 2015; 22: 123-4.
16. O'Donnell JN, Venkatesan N, Manek M, Rhodes NJ, Scheetz MH. Visual and absorbance analyses of admixtures containing vancomycin and piperacillin-tazobactam at commonly used concentrations. Am J Health-Syst Pharm 2016; 73: 241-6.
17. Vancomycin hydrochloride. In: IV index [internet]. Trissel's 2 clinical pharmaceutics database (parenteral compatibility). Ann Arbour, MI: Merative. Accessed 10/01/2023.

The Australian Injectable Drugs Handbook 9th ed. Abbotsford, Vic:
The Society of Hospital Pharmacists of Australia, July 2023.

Australian Injectable Drugs Handbook 9th Edition 565

PART **2**

SKILLS DEEPENING

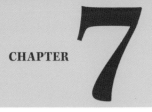

7 PAEDIATRIC CALCULATIONS

Introduction

Medication administration is very different when the person receiving the medicine is a child. Medicines need to be titrated accurately for these clients, according to their diagnosis, age and size. Children of certain ages can vary hugely in terms of weight and proportions and, as such, medication regimens need to be tailored to suit the individual. The majority of drug mistakes in paediatrics are due to calculation errors. It is important to remember that the person administering the medication is responsible for checking the dose that is ordered.

Paediatric medication doses can be calculated on a range of variables, from a combination of height and weight, age, body surface area (BSA) and as a proportion of the adult dose. The most common way of calculating a medication dose is as dose per kilogram. This concept was introduced in Chapter 5.

Dose per kilogram

The most common method used for prescribing paediatric medicine is as a dose per kilogram of body weight. Many of the major children's hospitals produce handbooks that give a recommended dose per kilogram for a range of medicines. The clinical procedures of your place of employment need to be followed to decide which handbook is used. Please note that for medications prescribed for children up to 16 years old, it is important to remember that the person administering the medication is responsible for checking that the **correct dose has been ordered by checking the child's weight and policies/guidelines for administration**.

The weight recorded for the child is best measured when the child is wearing little to no clothing. Clothing and nappies can add weight that can lead to an inadvertent medication overdose.

FORMULA 4 – DOSE PER KILOGRAM

$$\text{Dose to be given} = \text{recommended dose (mg/kg)} \times \text{weight (kg)}$$

Where:
'recommended dose/kg' has been prescribed or recommended in a drug handbook as the dose for children (e.g. *Australian Medicines Handbook* or a hospital handbook).

Many doses of medication are expressed as a total dose per day. This needs to be divided by the number of doses that have been prescribed by the doctor.

WORKED EXAMPLE 7.1

A child is ordered paracetamol for a fever. The recommended dosage for paracetamol is 15 mg/kg/dose 4–6 hourly. The child weighs 15 kg.

Dose to be given (mg) = recommended dose (mg/kg)
$$\times \text{ weight (kg)}$$

$$\text{Dose} = 15 \text{ mg/kg} \times 15 \text{ kg}$$
$$= 225 \text{ mg}$$

Formula method

$$\text{Dose} = \frac{\text{strength required}}{\text{stock strength}} \times \text{volume}$$

$$\text{Dose} = \frac{225 \text{ mg}}{48 \text{ mg}} \times 1 \text{ mL}$$

Dose = 4.68 mL

We would round this dose up to 4.7 mL.

Therefore we need to give the child 225 mg of paracetamol per dose.

Paracetamol is available in a strength of 48 mg/1 mL. Using the formula and methods described in Chapter 5, how much paracetamol should be given in each dose?

Proportion method

If we have: 48 mg = 1 mL
Then we want: 225 mg = x mL

> Ensure you put the same units on the same side of the equation (i.e. here both equations have mg on the left side).

Cross-multiply: 48 mg = 1 mL

225 mg = x mL

> Multiply everything diagonally (i.e. 48 × x = 48x and 225 × 1 = 225).

So: $48x = 225 \text{ mg}$

Solve for x: $\dfrac{48x}{48} = \dfrac{225 \text{ mg}}{48}$

> Divide both sides by 48 in order to get x by itself.

$$x = 4.68 \text{ mL}$$

We would round this up to 4.7 mL.

For the following activities, calculate:

a the dose to be given in mg

b the volume of the medicine to be administered.

1 A 6 kg child is prescribed ondansetron 0.15 mg/kg 8 hourly for nausea. Ondansetron is available in strength of 2 mg/mL.

2 A 7.5 kg child is prescribed chloral hydrate for sedation for a neuro-imaging procedure at a dose of 8 mg/kg/dose. Chloral hydrate is stocked in a 500 mg/5 mL bottle.

3 An 11 kg child is prescribed chlorpromazine. The order is for 0.5 mg/kg/dose. Chlorpromazine is available in a strength of 25 mg/5 mL.

Body surface area

Body surface area (BSA) may be used to calculate medication or fluid replacement for a client. This is particularly important when administering chemotherapy and when treating clients with burns. The BSA can be estimated by using a body surface nomogram (Figure 7.1) or by using the Mosteller formula (also referred to as the Mosteller equation). Using the equation is the most accurate method of calculating BSA, especially since most institutions have discontinued use of the nomogram due to errors with accuracy.

FORMULA 16 – BODY SURFACE AREA (BSA) USING THE MOSTELLER FORMULA

The calculation of BSA using the equation needs to be done using a calculator that has a function to calculate the square root.

The BSA calculations that are given in this text are obtained by multiplying the height by the weight. This answer is then divided by 3600. Following this, enter the $\sqrt{\ }$ key. This will give you the client's BSA in square metres.

$$BSA\ (m^2) = \sqrt{\frac{height\ (cm) \times weight\ (kg)}{3600}}$$

FIGURE 7.1 West Nomogram

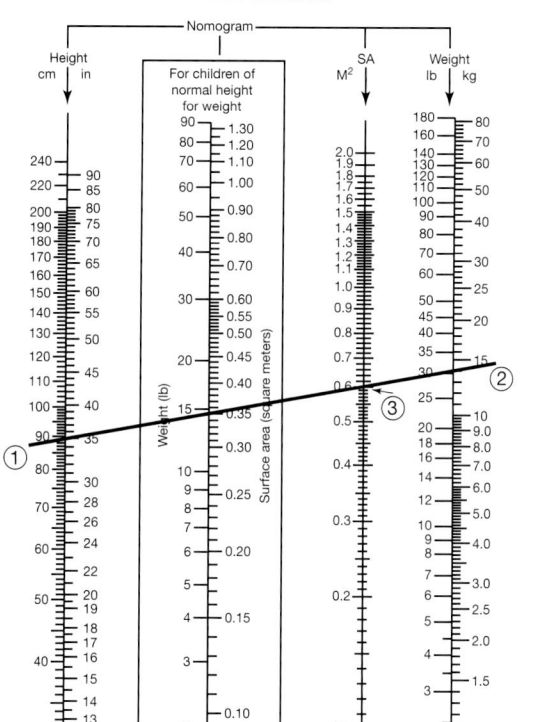

Body surface area (BSA) is determined by drawing a straight line from the client's height (1) in the far left column to his or her weight (2) in the far right column. Intersection of the line with surface area (SA) column (3) is the estimated BSA (m²). For infants and children of normal height and weight, BSA may be estimated from weight alone by referring to the enclosed area.

For a child of normal height for weight, the BSA can be determined on the West Nomogram using the weight alone. Notice the enclosed column to the center left. Normal height and weight standards can be found on pediatric growth and development charts.

Caution: To use the normal column on the West Nomogram, you must be familiar with normal height and weight standards for children. If you are unsure, use both height and weight to estimate BSA. Do not guess.

© Kliegman, R.M., Stanton, B.M.D, St. Geme, J., Schor, N. & Behrman, R.E. (2011). *Nelson textbook of pediatrics* [19th edn]. Philadelphia: Saunders (Elsevier). Reprinted with permission.

Nicholas is a 13-year-old boy who weighs 56 kg and is 164 cm high.
Work out his BSA using **Formula 16**.

$$\text{BSA (m}^2) = \sqrt{\frac{\text{ht(cm)} \times \text{wt(kg)}}{3600}}$$

$$\text{BSA (m}^2) = \sqrt{\frac{164 \times 56}{3600}}$$

$$= \sqrt{\frac{9184}{3600}}$$

$$= \sqrt{2.55}$$

$$= 1.60 \text{ m}^2$$

The answer from the calculation should be checked with the
West Nomogram.

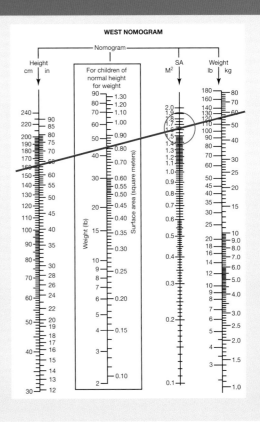

WORKED EXAMPLE 7.3

Christopher is an 11-year-old boy who weighs 44 kg and is 142 cm high. Work out his BSA using Formula 16.

$$\text{BSA (m}^2) = \sqrt{\frac{\text{ht(cm)} \times \text{wt(kg)}}{3600}}$$

$$\text{BSA (m}^2) = \sqrt{\frac{\text{ht(cm)} \times \text{wt(kg)}}{3600}}$$

$$= \sqrt{\frac{142 \times 44}{3600}}$$

$$= \sqrt{\frac{6248}{3600}}$$

$$= \sqrt{1.735}$$

$$= 1.32 \text{ m}^2$$

The answer from the calculation should be checked with the West Nomogram.

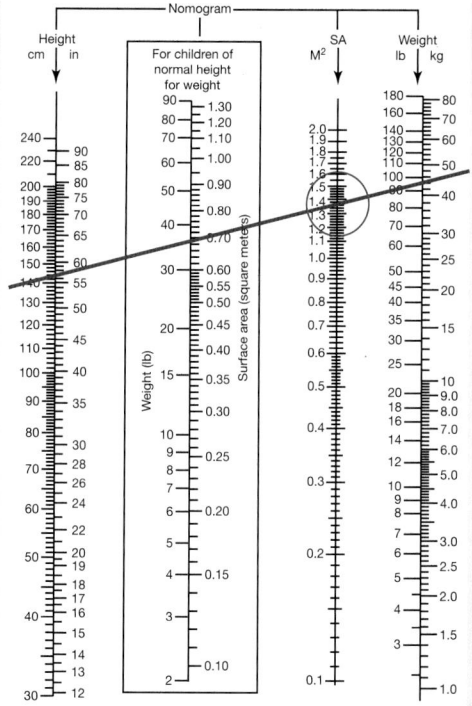

WEST NOMOGRAM

FIGURE 7.2 Ceftriaxone information

ACTIVITY 7.2

1   Emma is a 7-year-old girl whose weight has been recorded as 20 kg and height as 120 cm. Using the formula given, work out Emma's BSA. Compare this figure using the nomogram to check your answer.

2   Sam is an 8-month-old child with a recorded weight of 5.4 kg and a length of 58 cm. Work out Sam's BSA.

3   Annabel is 2 years old. She weighs 13 kg and is 90 cm high. Using the given formula, work out Annabel's BSA and check your answer using the nomogram.

Displacement values (powder volumes) when reconstituting powdered IV medications

When reconstituting medication from a powder to a liquid, the calculation of the volume required for the liquid is of utmost importance. The resultant volume will give an accurate dose per millilitre. Guidelines are available on the side of the packaging, in paediatric/intravenous drug resources or on the prescribing information leaflet. An example of this is given in Figure 7.2, for the antibiotic ceftriaxone.

cefTRIAXONE

BRAND NAME	CEFTRIAXONE AFT, VIATRIS
DRUG CLASS	Cephalosporin antibiotic
AVAILABILITY	Vial contains 0.5 g, 1 g or 2 g of ceftriaxone as ceftriaxone sodium. Each 1 g contains 3.6 mmol of sodium.[1]
WARNING	This is a cephalosporin (beta-lactam antibiotic). If the patient has a history of hypersensitivity to penicillins and/or cephalosporins, check with the treating team that allergy status has been considered.
pH	6–8 when reconstituted[1]
PREPARATION	**For IM use:**
	Reconstitute the 0.5 g vial with 2 mL and the 1 g vial with 3.5 mL of lidocaine 1%.[1] Reconstitute to 350 mg/mL for IM use in children.[2] (For the AFT 1 g vial use 2.3 mL). Solutions reconstituted with lidocaine must not be injected intravenously.[1]
	For IV use:
	Reconstitute the 0.5 g vial with 5 mL and the 1 g with 10 mL of water for injections, or 10–20 mL of sodium chloride 0.9%.[1,3]
	Reconstitute the 2 g vial with 40 mL of a compatible infusion fluid.[1]
	For the urgent treatment of critically unwell patients (e.g. sepsis), reconstitute the 2 g vial with 20 mL of water for injections or sodium chloride 0.9%.[3]
	Powder volume (AFT brand) 500 mg – 0.3 mL, 1 g – 0.6 mL, 2g – 1.1 mL[4]
	The solution is slightly opalescent and light yellow to amber. The solution may darken with storage but can still be used.[1]
STABILITY	Vial: store below 25 °C. Protect from light.[1]
	Reconstituted solution: stable for 6 hours below 25 °C and 24 hours at 2 to 8 °C.[1]
	If reconstituted with lidocaine for IM use, use immediately.
	Infusion solution: stable for 24 hours below 25 °C and 24 hours at 2 to 8 °C.[5]
	For CoPAT: solutions up to 40 mg/mL are stable for 24 hours below 25 °C.[6,7] There is no information about stability above 25 °C.
	Infusion solutions prepared in a sterile production unit are stable for more than 7 days at 2 to 8 °C.[5]
ADMINISTRATION	
IM injection	Suitable for adults and children. Inject into the gluteal muscle.[1] The ventrogluteal site is preferred. Divide the dose and give into the right and left side if required.[1]
SUBCUT infusion	Has been given by subcutaneous infusion over 30 minutes to 2 hours in patients with limited venous access.[8,9]

>>

IV injection	For doses up to 1 g, inject over 2 to 4 minutes.[1] Give doses of more than 1 g by IV infusion. In the urgent treatment of critically unwell patients (e.g. sepsis), a 2 g dose can be injected over 5 minutes.[3] See SPECIAL NOTES
IV infusion	Dilute the dose in approximately 40 mL of a compatible fluid and infuse over at least 30 minutes.[1] See SPECIAL NOTES
IV use for infants and children	Dilute to 40 mg/mL or weaker and infuse over 30 minutes. May be diluted to 40 mg/mL and injected over 5 minutes.[1,2] See SPECIAL NOTES

148 Australian Injectable Drugs Handbook 9th Edition

The Australian Injectable Drugs Handbook 9th ed. Abbotsford, Vic: The Society of Hospital Pharmacists of Australia; July 2023.

Powdered medications need to be reconstituted with a diluent (usually water or 0.9% saline for injection) before use. In order to calculate how many mg per mL are in the resultant solution, the displacement value (powder volume) needs to be taken into account. Since a child's dose is often smaller than an adult's dose, only a small portion of the vial is usually used – it is then possible to take a small amount of the reconstituted vial and know precisely the dose of medicine in the withdrawn amount.

For example, when 10 mL water is added to a powder, the resultant volume may be greater than 10 mL, making it harder to withdraw an accurate dose. Think of when powder is added to milk (i.e. adding cocoa or flavoured powder) – the fluid level rises, and this is the same with medicines.

In order to add the correct amount of diluent, the 'displacement value' (or powder volume) must be taken into account. This amount can be known from the drug resources/information leaflets. For example, ceftazidime 1 g has a displacement value of 1.1 mL (i.e. 1 g = 1.1 mL). In order to draw up a dose of 400 mg, it is easier to make the resultant solution up to 10 mL total (i.e. 100 mg per mL). To do this, we subtract 1.1 mL from 10 mL to establish that we need to add 8.9 mL diluent (water for injection) to the vial, then mix. Of this total solution, 4 mL would contain 400 mg of ceftazidime.

Some powdered medicines have a negligible displacement value so that when the powder is mixed with the diluent the total volume does not change, so no further calculation is required. For example, erythromycin has a negligible displacement value so a full 10 mL of diluent is added to a 1 g vial to give 100 mg/mL solution.

Displacement values may also be given in a table form on the drug information leaflet. For an example of this, refer to Figure 7.2.

A medication chart may state a dose of 700 mg of ceftriaxone IV. The vial of the antibiotic available is 1 g. After consulting the reconstitution table, it is simple to work out that if you reconstitute the vial with 9.6 mL of water for injection, you have a result of 100 mg/mL. The remaining 0.4 mL is the volume of the powder.

For a dose of 700 mg, you will therefore withdraw 7 mL of the reconstituted solution.

Worked example 7.4 illustrates this for the antibiotic cefalotin.

WORKED EXAMPLE 7.4

Order: cefalotin 700 mg IV

A vial of cefalotin has a powder volume/displacement volume of 1 g = 0.4 mL.

How do you reconstitute this vial so you can deliver this?

10 mL water for injection (WFI) − 0.4 mL (powder volume) = 9.6 mL WFI required.

9.6 mL WFI gives 100 mg/1 mL

Therefore, you would withdraw 7 mL of the reconstituted solution to give 700 mg.

ACTIVITY 7.3

Solve the following reconstitution problems to give a total of 10 mL solution:

a Determine the amount of diluent required.

b Determine what volume of the medication you will administer.

1 Order: piperacillin 1.5 g IV
Available: 2 g vial of piperacillin
Powder volume: 0.7 mL/g

2 Order: flucloxacillin 150 mg IV
Available: 250 mg vial of flucloxacillin
Powder volume: 0.2 mL/250 mg

3 Order: chloramphenicol 750 mg IV
Available: 1 g vial of chloramphenicol
Powder volume: 1.2 mL/g

Practical calculations

WORKED EXAMPLE 7.5

CLINICAL CASE STUDY

Christopher Wines is a 12-year-old child who has been admitted into a paediatric ward for treatment for tonsillitis requiring antibiotics and analgesia. He has had a past history of several admissions for tonsillitis and severe otitis media. He weighs 40 kg and his height was recorded as being 152 cm. He is febrile at 39.8 °C.

It is now 1400 hrs on 25 April. Refer to Christopher's medication chart and work through the '10 steps for safe use of a medication chart'.

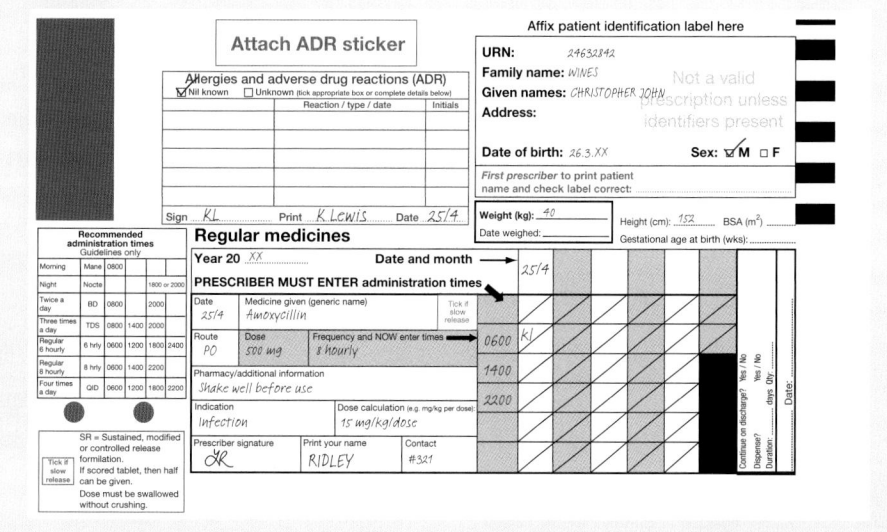

Date	Medicine (print generic name)		Tick if slow release	
25/4	ceftriaxone			
Route	**Dose**	Frequency and NOW enter times →		1700
IV	2 grams	daily		
Pharmacy/additional information				
Limit 2 g/dose				
Indication		Dose calculation (eg. mg/kg per dose)		
Infection		50 mg/kg/dose		
Prescriber signature	Print your name	Contact/pager		
JR	RIDLEY	# 321		

Continue on discharge? Yes / No
Dispense? Yes / No
Duration: ......days Qty: ......
Pager: ...... Date: ......

Affix patient identification label here

URN: 24632842
Family name: WINES
Given names: CHRISTOPHER JOHN
Address:
Date of birth: 26.3.XX
Sex: ☑ M ☐ F

Not a valid Prescription unless Identifiers present

First prescriber to print patient name and check label correct: ......

Attach ADR sticker

See front page for details

As required PRN medicines

Weight (kg): 40
Date weighed: ......

Ward/unit: 4 C

Date	Medicine given (generic name)			Date	
25/4	paracetamol				
Route	**Dose**	Hourly frequency	Max PRN dose/24 hrs	Time	
PO	600 mg	4 hrly **PRN**	4 g/24 hr		
Pharmacy/additional information				**Dose**	
Antipyretic					
Indication		Dose calculation (eg. mg/kg per dose)		Route	
Antipyretic		15 mg/kg			
Prescriber signature	Print your name		Contact/pager	Sign	
JVL	RIDLEY		# 321		

Continue on discharge? Yes / No
Dispense? Yes / No
Duration: ......days Qty: ......
Date: ......

Work out Christopher's BSA.

$$\text{BSA (m}^2) = \sqrt{\frac{\text{height} \times \text{weight}}{3600}}$$

$$= \sqrt{\frac{152 \times 40}{3600}}$$

$$= \sqrt{\frac{6080}{3600}}$$

$$= \sqrt{1.68}$$

$$= 1.30 \text{ m}^2$$

>>

>>

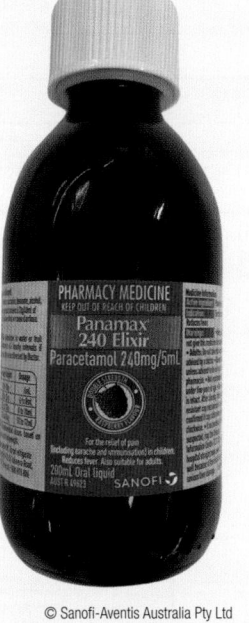

PRESCRIPTION ONLY MEDICINE
KEEP OUT OF REACH OF CHILDREN

Amoxycillin Sandoz®

amoxicillin trihydrate 250 mg/5 mL

powder for oral suspension
100 mL (when mixed)

1 bottle

Sugar-Free

Each 5 mL of reconstituted
suspension contains
amoxicillin 250 mg
(as trihydrate)

AUST R 93720

SANDOZ A Novartis Division

© Sandoz Pty Ltd 2019   © Sanofi-Aventis Australia Pty Ltd

In order to calculate what medicine doses are now due,
let's review the '10 steps for safe use of a medication chart'
as outlined in previous chapters.

SAFETY ⚠️

10 STEPS FOR SAFE USE OF A MEDICATION CHART

Step 1   Scan medication chart to ensure the prescription(s)
meet legal requirements and are able to be used.

Step 2   Check which medicines are due/available to
administer now.

Step 3   Check for any interactions or contraindications. If
medicines have a risk of serious adverse effects, then
ensure you are able to monitor/manage these safely.

Step 4   Check that the dosage and route are appropriate for
the client's condition.

Step 5   Assess the client to see if the medicine(s) are
suitable for them at this time. Ensure no allergies or
contraindications to this medicine.

Step 6   Think about this dose – is it logical (e.g. you would not
expect to give more than a couple of tablets or a few
mL out of a bottle)?

Step 7   Convert all measurements to the same units, then
perform dosage calculations using either the formula
or the proportions method. This ensures the correct
amount of medicine is given.

Step 8   Administer the medicine following the '7 rights',
ensuring the client or their carer understands and
consents to this.

Step 9   Sign/document the medicine as administered on the
appropriate charts.

Step 10   Assess the client for any adverse effects.

WORKED EXAMPLE – ANSWERS

Step 1	✓	All prescriptions on this medicine chart are complete and meet legal requirements.
Step 2	✓	Two of the medicines on this chart are due now at 1400 hrs.
Step 3	✓	No significant interactions/precautions are noted.
Step 4	✓	Dosage and routes seem appropriate for paediatric client.
Step 5	✓	The client has no allergies and seems stable for these medicines.
Step 6	→	Let's work out these dose calculations as shown below …

AMOXYCILLIN

Order: Christopher has been prescribed amoxycillin 500 mg 8 hourly.

Available: Amoxycillin is available as a liquid in a stock strength of 250 mg in 5 mL.

Calculate the dosage to be given.

Formula method

$$\text{Volume required} = \frac{\text{strength required}}{\text{stock strength}} \times \text{volume of stock solution}$$

$$= \frac{500 \text{ mg}}{250 \text{ mg}} \times 5 \text{ mL}$$

$$= \frac{2 \text{ mg}}{1 \text{ mg}} \times 5 \text{ mL}$$

$$\text{Dose} = 10 \text{ mL}$$

Proportions method

If we have: 250 mg = 5 mL
Then we want: 500 mg = x mL

> Ensure you put the same units on the same side of the equation (i.e. here both equations have mg on the left side).

Cross-multiply: 250 mg = 5 mL

500 mg = x mL

> Multiply everything diagonally ($250 \times x = 250x$ and $5 \times 500 = 2500$).

So: $250x = 2500$

Solve for x: $\dfrac{250x}{250} = \dfrac{2500}{250}$

$x = 10$ mL

> Divide both sides by 250 to get x by itself.

>>

>>

Administer...

Ensure that you have washed your hands before administration. Shake the bottle to evenly distribute medicine in the liquid and then draw up 10 mL of amoxycillin in a syringe to administer directly into the client's mouth with the syringe.

PARACETAMOL

Paracetamol is available as 240 mg in 5 mL. If you divide 240 by 5, then the concentration of this solution is 48 mg/mL.

Formula method

$$\text{Volume required} = \frac{\text{strength required}}{\text{stock strength}} \times \text{volume of stock solution}$$

$$= \frac{600 \text{ mg}}{48 \text{ mg}} \times 1$$

$$= \frac{600}{48}$$

$$= 12.5 \text{ mL}$$

Proportions method

If we have: 48 mg = 1 mL
Then we want: 600 mg = x mL

Cross-multiply: 48 mg = 1 mL

600 mg = x mL

So: $48x = 600$

Solve for x: $\dfrac{48x}{48} = \dfrac{600}{48}$

$x = 12.5$ mL

Ensure you have the same units on the same side of the equation (i.e. here both equations have mg on the left side).

Multiply everything diagonally ($48 \times x = 48x$ and $1 \times 600 = 600$).

Divide both sides by 48 to get x by itself.

Administer…

If paracetamol is required, draw 12.5 mL in a syringe and administer to the child directly into the mouth.

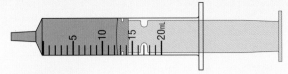

🔍 CLINICAL CASE STUDY (CONTINUED)

It is now 1700 hrs on 25 April.

Christopher remains febrile, and sensitivities return from pathology stating that his antibiotic therapy needs to be changed to ceftriaxone. He is cannulated in order to deliver the antibiotic via IV access.

Calculate the amount given to Christopher from a reconstituted solution.

CEFTRIAXONE

Refer to the dosage information for ceftriaxone given earlier (see Figure 7.2).

Order: Ceftriaxone 2 g IV
Available: A 2 g vial of ceftriaxone.
Add 19.2 mL normal saline to obtain a concentration of 100 mg/mL.

Formula method

$$\text{Volume required} = \frac{\text{strength required}}{\text{stock strength}} \times \frac{\text{volume of stock}}{\text{solution}}$$

$$= \frac{2000}{100} \times 1$$

$$= 20 \text{ mL}$$

Proportions method

If we have:	100 mg = 1 mL
Then we want:	2000 mg = x

> Ensure you put the same units on the same side of the equation (i.e. here both equations have mg on the left side).

Cross-multiply: 100 mg = 1 mL

2000 mg = x

> Multiply everything diagonally (i.e. 100 × x = 100x and 1 × 2000 = 2000).

So: $100x = 2000$

Solve for x: $\dfrac{100x}{100} = \dfrac{2000}{100}$

> Divide both sides by 100 to get x by itself.

$x = 20$ mL

>>

ACTIVITY 7.4

CLINICAL CASE STUDY

Ben Branch is a 7-year-old boy who was playing at the local playground with his friends. He came to hospital following a fall from the climbing bars a few hours ago and has just been admitted to the ward with a fractured ulna and radius.

He has a past medical history of autism spectrum disorder and asthma, but does not tolerate use of metered dose inhaler so needs to have nebulised salbutamol. He has no known allergies. He has a medication chart that gives him his bronchodilators, analgesics and antibiotics post-surgery for pinning his fractures.

It is now 0800 hrs on 25 April. Refer to Ben Branch's medication chart and work through the '10 steps for safe use of a medication chart'.

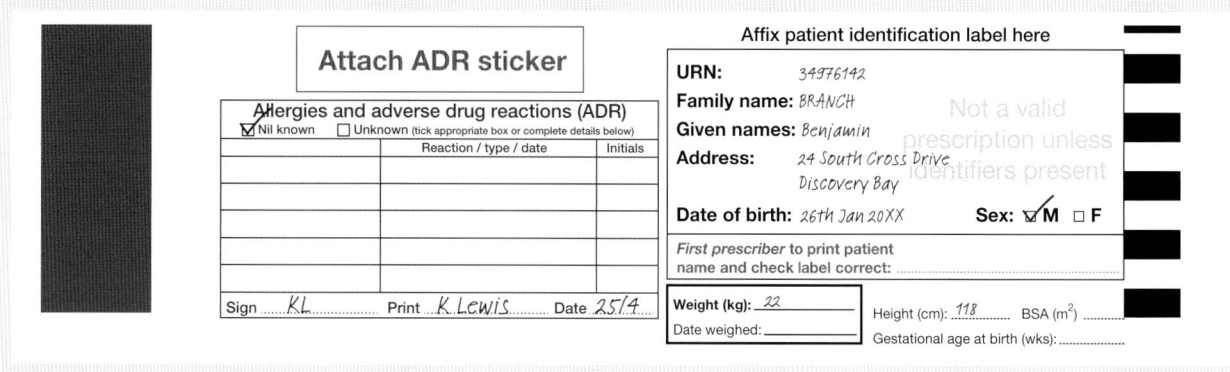

(continued)

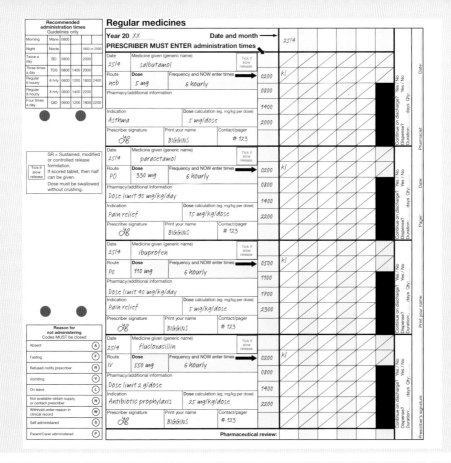

>>

PRESCRIPTION ONLY MEDICINE
KEEP OUT OF REACH OF CHILDREN

Salbutamol inhalation ampoules 5 mg/2.5 mL

30 ampoules

Each ampoule with 2.5 mL contains salbutamol
sulphate equivalent to salbutamol 5 mg

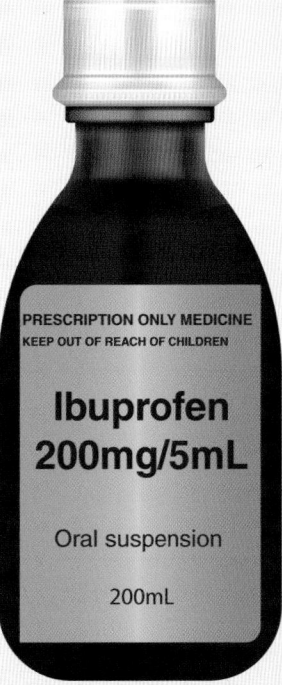

PRESCRIPTION ONLY MEDICINE
KEEP OUT OF REACH OF CHILDREN

Ibuprofen
200mg/5mL

Oral suspension

200mL

© Reckitt Benckiser. Nurofen for Children 5-12 Years
contains 200 mg ibuprofen per 5 mL. Label current
as on 11 June 2019. Always refer to pack for up-to-
date dosing instructions.

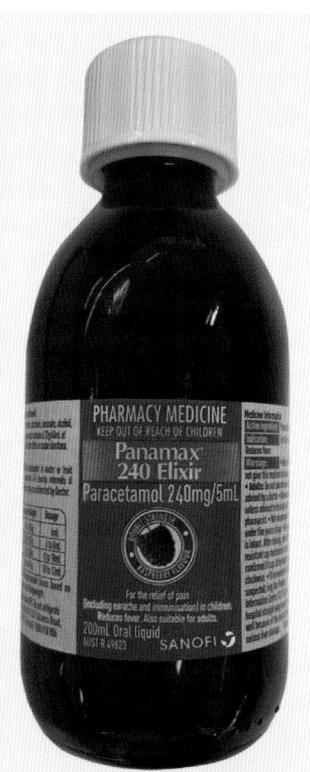

PHARMACY MEDICINE
KEEP OUT OF REACH OF CHILDREN
Panamax
240 Elixir
Paracetamol 240mg/5mL

For the relief of pain
(Including earache and immunisation) in children.
Reduces fever. Also suitable for adults.
200mL Oral liquid
AUST R 49623

SANOFI

© Sanofi-Aventis Australia Pty Ltd

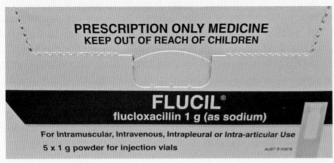

© Aspen Pharmacare

1 Calculate Ben's BSA.
2 Using the formulae, calculate the dosages for the medicines that are due. (For a concentration of 100 mg/mL of flucloxacillin, add sterile water for injection to the vial to a total of 10 mL.)

Introduction

Medication administration in maternity care is a process that needs to consider both the mother's and child's welfare. Most medications will cross the placenta; therefore, all medicines in Australia are given a risk category according to any known short- or long-term risks to the fetus/baby. This aids in assessing the risk versus benefits of certain drugs in pregnancy. This applies to drugs for a breastfeeding mother also. Following administration of medicine to the mother during labour, the neonate may take two to three days to clear the metabolites of that medicine (Jordan, 2010).

The midwife has a role in managing medication administration during the pregnancy, labour and postnatal period for mothers and babies. Knowledge of what medications are recommended, dose, route and under what circumstances in this period is part of a midwife's scope of practice. Certain medications are allowed to be given by a midwife under the guidelines of the standing orders without a doctor's signature. Ensuring up-to-date knowledge of any changes to standing orders is imperative for safe practice.

During pregnancy, standing orders include recommended vaccinations, certain vitamins and minerals and Rh (D) immunoglobulin (Anti-D) 625 IU. During labour, standing orders include analgesia and antiemetics. In the postnatal period, standing orders include analgesia and Anti-D as indicated. For the newborn, midwives have the responsibility for administering phytomenadione (Vitamin K) and hepatitis B vaccination. It is important to note that consent from the woman is necessary before administration of any medication to herself or the baby.

Women with pre-existing medical conditions or conditions that may emerge as complications during pregnancy may need their medications managed by midwives during any admission. The midwife can also ensure a woman understands what medication she is taking and for what reason to help reassure her of the safety of taking the medication and the risk that not taking this may pose to her and/or her baby. This includes medication that may be recommended but not limited to conditions such as urinary tract infections, pregnancy-induced hypertension, gestational diabetes, premature labour and conditions that may indicate induction of labour.

Midwives will work with a variety of women requiring different levels of intervention and care. A midwife needs to have the skills to deal with the administration of medicines in critical situations when medical assistance may not be available or, at best, only available over the telephone.

Labour and birth

The majority of medicines used during labour and birth are analgesics, regional or local anaesthetics and anti-emetics. Oxytocics are commonly used to induce or augment labour (in the presence of ruptured membranes) and are recommended routinely (10 units at the end of the second stage of labour), either intravenously or intramuscularly to prevent postpartum haemorrhage. Oxytocics are also given when the cause of a postpartum haemorrhage is established as a poorly contracted uterus.

The use of oral medicine in labour is limited, as the pharmacokinetics of medicines may be altered during labour and delivery due to the potential for delayed gastric emptying in some women. Delayed gastric emptying can also lead to nausea and vomiting. As a result, parenteral routes for medication administration are more commonly used. An exception is the routine use of an antacid prior to an emergency caesarean section.

Pharmacological methods of pain relief are determined by the mother's wishes, the availability of different forms of pain relief, the situation under which the pain relief is being given and the availability of appropriate prescribers to order and deliver alternative forms of pain relief, such as spinal or epidural medications.

The most common pain relief during labour is administered via inhalation in the form of nitrous oxide and oxygen (RANZCOG, 2016). For effective analgesia, nitrous oxide and oxygen concentrations (commonly 40% N_2 : 60% O_2) need to be titrated according to the individual's needs (Likis et al., 2014). Despite its relative safety, the use of nitrous oxide must still be monitored by the midwife to manage any nausea and/or lightheadedness by increasing the percentage of O_2 to N_2.

Narcotics such as morphine (5–10 mg) or fentanyl provide stronger pain relief. Individual hospital practice tends to determine preference for the type of narcotic recommended in labour. Midwifery standing orders are usually for intramuscular or subcutaneous injection only, but intravenous injection is also a common method of delivery of this form of pain relief.

Regional anaesthesia in the form of epidural (injection of local anaesthetic into the epidural space) for labour or spinal (anaesthetic into the subarachnoid space) for caesareans are administered by an anaesthetist. Midwives take responsibility for delivering the medication, usually via a syringe pump, both during labour and, if required, after caesarean.

Local anaesthetics injected into the perineal tissue (muscle and skin) provide short-term pain relief before cutting an episiotomy and for suturing perineal tears and/or episiotomy.

Calculation of the volume of an injection to be given is relatively straightforward, and is based on Formula 5.

CHAPTER 8

FORMULA 5 – DOSAGE CALCULATION: TABLETS AND LIQUIDS

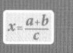

$$Dose = \frac{strength\ required}{stock\ strength} \times volume$$

You must ensure that the strength required and stock strength are both in the same units (convert to the smaller units if necessary).

Where:
- 'strength required' is the required dose
- 'stock strength' is the concentration of the stock you have ready to administer from
- 'volume' is the amount related to the 'stock strength' (e.g. if you have 5 mg in one tablet, the stock strength is 5 mg and the volume [quantity] is 1 tablet. If you have a liquid concentration 10 mg/2 mL, then the stock strength is 10 mg and the volume is 2 mL).

Local anaesthetics

In midwifery practice, local anaesthetics provide short-term pain relief. There are several different routes for local anaesthetics used in midwifery:
- topical therapy (e.g. before cannulation)
- intradermally or subcutaneously (e.g. for suturing or managing perineal pain from traumatic tearing).

CLINICAL CASE STUDY

Fiona Thomas is a 32-year-old primigravid woman who has gone into premature labour at 28 weeks gestation. Membranes are intact and she is contracting 3 in 10 minutes.

You are looking after her in the birth suite; she has been prescribed medication to stop her labour. The time is 0928 hrs.

Medicine chart no. _1_ **of** _1_

Facility/service: _Fairview Hospital_

Ward/unit: _Midwifery Unit_

Additional charts
- ☐ IV fluid
- ☐ Palliative care
- ☐ Bgl/insulin
- ☐ Chemotherapy
- ☐ Acute pain
- ☐ Iv heparin
- ☐ Other

Once only and nurse initiated medicines and pre-medications

Date prescribed	Medicine (print generic name)	Route	Dose	Date/time of dose	Prescriber/Nurse Initiator (NI) Signature	Print your name	Given by	Time given	Pharm:
23/8	Nifedipine	PO	20 mg	23/8 0930	J Grace	GRACE			
	If contractions continue, follow with next order after 30 mins								
23/8	Nifedipine	PO	20 mg	23/8 1000	J Grace	GRACE			
	If contractions persist, follow with following order after 30 mins								
23/8	Nifedipine	PO	20 mg	23/8 1030	J Grace	GRACE			

In order to calculate what medicine doses are to be given, let's review the '10 steps for safe use of a medication chart'.

>>

CHAPTER 8

>>

SAFETY

10 STEPS FOR SAFE USE OF A MEDICATION CHART

Step 1 Scan medication chart to ensure the prescription(s) are legal and are able to be used.

Step 2 Check which medicines are due/available to administer now.

Step 3 Check for any interactions or contraindications. If medicines have a risk of serious adverse effects, then ensure you are able to monitor/manage these safely.

Step 4 Check that the dosage and route are appropriate for the client's condition.

Step 5 Assess the client to see if the medicine(s) are suitable for them at this time. Ensure no allergies or contraindications to this medicine.

Step 6 Think about this dose – is it logical (e.g. you would not expect to give more than a couple of tablets or a few mL out of a bottle)?

Step 7 Convert all measurements to the same units and then perform dosage calculations using either the formula or the proportions method. This ensures the correct amount of medicine is given.

Step 8 Administer the medicine following the '7 rights', ensuring the client understands and consents to this.

Step 9 Sign/document the medicine as administered on the appropriate charts.

Step 10 Assess the client for any adverse effects.

So let's now work through these steps and calculate the doses.

WORKED EXAMPLE – ANSWERS

Step 1	✓	All prescriptions on this medicine chart are complete and meet legal requirements.
Step 2	✓	There is one medicine on this chart due now.
Step 3	✓	No significant interactions/precautions are noted.
Step 4	✓	Dosage and routes are appropriate for this pregnant client.
Step 5	✓	The client has no allergies and has been assessed as being in a stable condition for these medicines.
Step 6	→	Let's work out these dose calculations as shown below …

NIFEDIPINE

Nifedipine is a calcium channel blocker that is effective in inhibiting premature uterine contractions. It has been found to have fewer adverse effects for both mother and baby than other tocolytic medications in a 2014 Cochrane Collection Systematic Review (Flenady et al., 2014). Nifedipine is given orally and it is available as a 20 mg tablet.

Formula method

$$\text{Dose} = \frac{\text{strength required}}{\text{stock strength}} \times \text{volume}$$

$$= \frac{20 \text{ mg}}{20 \text{ mg}}$$

$$= 1 \text{ tablet}$$

Proportions method

If we have:	20 mg nifedipine = 1 tablet
Then we want:	20 mg = x tablet

Ensure you put the same units on the same side of the equation (i.e. here both equations have mg on the left side).

Cross-multiply:

20 mg = 1 tablet

20 mg = x tablet

Multiply everything diagonally (i.e. 20 × x = 20x and 20 × 1 = 20).

So:

$$20x = 20$$

Solve for x:

$$\frac{20x}{20} = \frac{20}{20}$$

$$x = 1 \text{ tablet}$$

Divide both sides by 20 in order to get x by itself.

ACTIVITY 8.1

CLINICAL CASE STUDY

Clare Eloise is a 24-year-old multigravid woman (weighing 70 kg) who has been admitted to the birth suite in active labour. She has had a normal uncomplicated pregnancy and her labour is progressing well.

You are looking after her in the birth suite and are reviewing her medication chart. You find medication orders written on the chart.

1a Calculate how many of these medicines are appropriate to be administered.

Affix patient identification label here and overleaf

URN:	063421
Family name:	ELOISE
Given names:	CLARE
Address:	32 Pietty view RD
	Riverside
Date of birth:	26/4/XX **Sex:** ☐ M ☑ F

Not a valid prescription unless identifiers present

First prescriber to print patient name and check label correct: .... GRANT

Attach ADR sticker

See front page for details

**As required
PRN
medicines**

Year: 20 XX

Date 23/8	Medicine (print generic name) Fentanyl			Date													Continue on discharge? Yes / No	Dispense? Yes / No	days Qty....	Duration...
Route IV	Dose 35 microg	Hourly frequency 4/24 **PRN**	Max PRN dose/24 hrs 2 microg/kg	Time																
Indication Pain		Pharmacy		Dose																
				Route																
Prescriber signature J Grant	Print your name GRANT		Contact # 321	Sign																
Date 23/8	Medicine (print generic name) Metoclopramide			Date													Continue on discharge? Yes / No	Dispense? Yes / No	days Qty....	Duration...
Route IV	Dose 10 mg	Hourly frequency 6/24 **PRN**	Max PRN dose/24 hrs 0.5 mg/kg	Time																
Indication Nausea/vomiting		Pharmacy		Dose																
				Route																
Prescriber signature J Grant	Print your name GRANT		Contact # 321	Sign																

Clare goes on to giving birth quickly. The placenta and membranes follow within five minutes of the birth of the baby. It soon becomes apparent that she is having a postpartum haemorrhage.

You go to assist the primary midwife in managing this situation. You are asked to 'Give 0.25 mg of ergometrine IV right now!' The doctor also urgently requests oxytocin 40 units into a bag of Hartmanns solution 1000 mL to be run over 4 hours.

This is written on the medication chart on page 172.

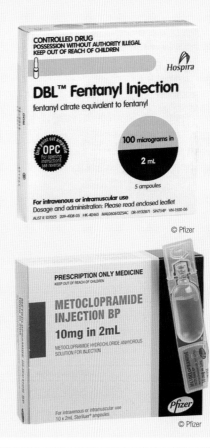

© Pfizer

© Pfizer

CHAPTER 8

>>

Medicine chart no. 1 of 1

Facility/service: _Fairview Hospital_

Ward/unit: _Midwifery Unit_

Additional charts

☐ IV fluid ☐ Bgl/insulin ☐ Acute pain ☐ Other
☐ Palliative care ☐ Chemotherapy ☐ Iv heparin

	Once only and nurse initiated medicines and pre-medications								
Date prescribed	Medicine (print generic name)	Route	Dose	Date/time of dose	Prescriber/Nurse Initiator (NI)		Given by	Time given	Pharmacy
					Signature	Print your name			
23/8	Oxytocin in 1000 mL Hartmanns	IV	40 units	stat over 4 hrs	J Grace	GRACE			
23/8	Ergometrine	IV	0.25 mg	STAT	J Grace	GRACE			

Ergometrine is available as an ampoule containing 500 micrograms in 1 mL. Oxytocin is available as 10 units/mL.

1b Calculate the volume of ergometrine to be given. Calculate the volume of oxytocin to be added to the Hartmanns solution, and the rate for the oxytocin infusion to be run.

PRESCRIPTION ONLY MEDICINE
KEEP OUT OF REACH OF CHILDREN

Oxytocin 10 IU/1mL
Solution for injection
IM or IV use only

5 × 1 mL ampoules

PRESCRIPTION ONLY MEDICINE
KEEP OUT OF REACH OF CHILDREN

Hospira

DBL™ Ergometrine Injection
ergometrine maleate

OPC
the patent cut ampoule
For immediate
instruction
see reverse

500 micrograms in **1 mL**

5 ampoules

For intramuscular or intravenous injection only
Dosage and administration: Please read enclosed leaflet
AUST R 58866   MAL19950195A   SIN2861P

© Pfizer

Clare's baby has been born with good Apgar scores and is now one hour old. You have been asked to attend to the baby and administer the Vitamin K injection (phytomenadione) that Clare had consented to prior to the baby's birth.

You find the medication chart and look at the medication orders.

1c Calculate the volume that would be given.

👶 Paediatric   **Medicine chart no.** _1_   **of** _1_

Facility/service: _Fairview Hospital_

Ward/unit: _Midwifery_

Additional charts
- ☐ IV fluid
- ☐ Inhalation
- ☐ BGL/insulin
- ☐ Palliative care
- ☐ Acute pain
- ☐ Chemotherapy
- ☐ IV heparin
- ☐ Other

					Prescriber/Nurse Initiator (NI)				
Once only medicines									
Date prescribed	Medicine (print generic name)	Route	Dose	Date/time of dose	Signature	Print your name	Given by	Time given	Pharmacy
23/8	Phytomenadione	IM	1 mg	23/8 1400	J Grant	GRANT			

PRESCRIPTION ONLY MEDICINE
KEEP OUT OF REACH OF CHILDREN

Phytomenadione 2 mg/0.2 mL

5 ampoules and 5 dispensers

Mixed micelles solutions for oral, intravenous or intramuscular administration

AUST R 71758

CHAPTER 6

CRITICAL CARE AND HIGH DEPENDENCY DOSAGE CALCULATIONS

Introduction

Critical care and high dependency clinical areas include the emergency department, operating theatre, post-anaesthetic care unit, intensive care unit, coronary care unit and cardiology areas. In general terms, dosage calculations in these areas follow the same basic principles as outlined in earlier chapters of this book; however, there may be some more complex calculations performed pertaining to infusions. Many of the medicines prescribed in these areas are highly potent and need to be titrated exactly to a client's condition; it is for this reason that calculations may be more complex (incorporating dose per minute and dose per body weight per minute). It is important to realise that healthcare settings are increasing in client complexity and therefore many of these calculations may also be applicable to some general ward areas, making it important for all health professionals to understand these calculations. The Australian Commission on Safety and Quality in Health Care identified the ongoing use of potentially dangerous abbreviations and dose expressions as one of the major causes of medication errors.

Therefore, the term 'microg' has replaced 'mcg' in best practice. However, some areas of the healthcare industry, such as critical care, still refer to micrograms as mcg, and therefore this term will be used in some parts of this chapter.

This chapter introduces the reader to calculating correct doses in units per minute (e.g. microg/min or mg/min), units per body weight per minute (e.g. microg/kg/min or mg/kg/min) and how to calculate volumes required for bolus infusion doses. This chapter also includes medication concentration calculations as these are needed to complete the additive labels required when infusions of many medicines are used.

General principles for solving calculations in units/min and units/body weight/min

As already discussed in previous chapters, infusion pumps typically only allow the health professional to set the rate (i.e. mL/h) and the total volume to be infused. Some medicines, however, are very potent and/or dangerous and these are often ordered in terms of the amount of medicine that the client receives per minute (microg/min or mg/min). Sometimes the medicines are ordered according to the client's body weight (e.g. microg/kg/min or mg/kg/min). Given that the infusion pump can usually only be input with the rate in terms of mL/h, calculations need to be performed to convert microg/min (or mg/min or microg/kg/min or mg/kg/min, depending on the medicine ordered) to mL/h.

The infusion may be prepared commercially, or by hospital pharmacists or by health professionals at the client's bedside. The way the infusion is made up is not relevant to the calculation of the dose (assuming the infusion has been made correctly). The key information that you need to discover is the overall concentration of the solution (e.g. 6 mg of noradrenaline in 100 mL of intravenous [IV] fluid). This is written either on the infusion flask itself (commercially prepared infusions) or on an approved infusion additive label (for infusions prepared by the pharmacy department or by health professionals in the clinical area). Then you need to establish the amount of medicine in 1 mL of the fluid (the type of fluid or medication is not relevant to performing the actual calculation).

Infusion calculations – units per minute (microg/min or mg/min)

The two key stages to solving microg/min (or mg/min) calculations are shown here.

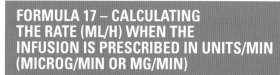

FORMULA 17 – CALCULATING THE RATE (ML/H) WHEN THE INFUSION IS PRESCRIBED IN UNITS/MIN (MICROG/MIN OR MG/MIN)

$x = \frac{a \cdot b}{c}$

Stage 1 Calculate rate in mL/min.
$$\text{Rate (mL/min)} = \frac{\text{strength required}}{\text{stock strength}} \times \text{volume}$$

Stage 2 Calculate flow rate in mL/h.
$$\text{Rate mL/h} = \text{mL/min} \times 60 \text{ min/h}$$

WORKED EXAMPLE 9.1

 CLINICAL CASE STUDY (MCG/MIN)

Aniela Gallina is an elderly woman requiring an adrenaline infusion for severe hypotension due to sepsis.

The prescriber has ordered an adrenaline infusion, which has just been made up by a registered nurse. Its concentration may be seen on the infusion label. The infusion rate needs to be set to 4 microg/min.

What do you need to do?

>>

>>

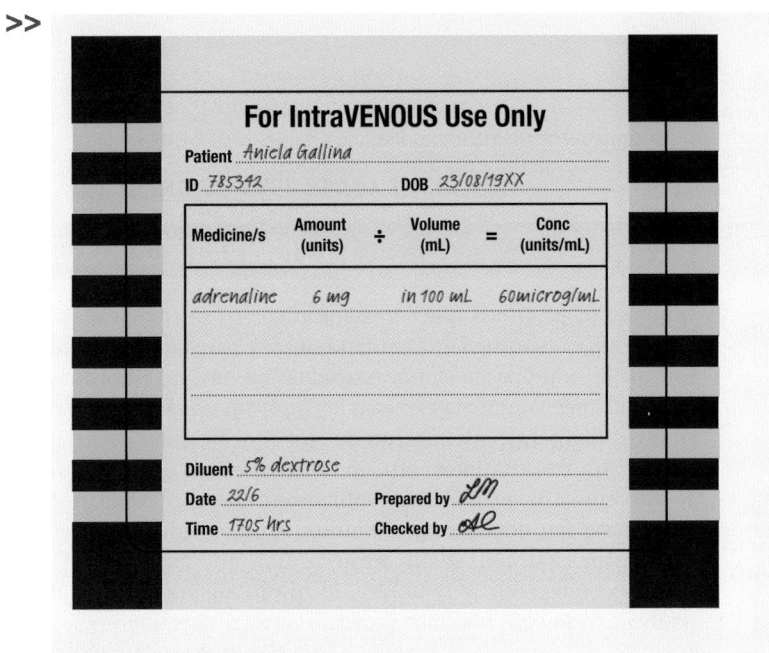

For IntraVENOUS Use Only

Patient _Aniela Gallina_

ID _785342_   DOB _23/08/19XX_

Medicine/s	Amount (units)	÷	Volume (mL)	=	Conc (units/mL)
adrenaline	6 mg		in 100 mL		60microg/mL

Diluent _5% dextrose_

Date _22/6_   Prepared by _LM_

Time _1705 hrs_   Checked by _AC_

Please refer to the '10 steps for safe use of a medication chart' before starting your calculations.

There are a few steps required in these sorts of calculations. It is important to remember that the 5% dextrose is a 'type' of intravenous fluid so the '5%' part may be ignored in this case (this is often a source of confusion for students).

Now let's follow the two stages to solving microg/min as detailed earlier.

STAGE 1 CALCULATE RATE IN ML/MIN

Formula method

We have 6 mg adrenaline in 100 mL fluid
(note: 6 mg = 6000 microg)

$$\text{Rate (mL/min)} = \frac{\text{strength required}}{\text{stock strength}} \times \text{volume}$$

$$= \frac{4 \text{ microg/min}}{6000 \text{ microg}} \times 100 \text{ mL}$$

$$= 0.067 \text{ mL/min}$$

Proportions method

If we have:	6 mg (6000 mcg)	= 100 mL
	adrenaline	5% dextrose
Then we want:	4 microg/min	= x mL

> Ensure you put the same units on the same side of the equation (i.e. here both equations have microg on the left side).

Cross-multiply:

$$6000 \text{ microg} = 100 \text{ mL}$$
$$4 \text{ microg/min} = x \text{ mL}$$

> Multiply everything diagonally
> (i.e. 6000 × x = 6000x
> and 100 × 4 = 400)

So:

$$6000x = 400$$

Solve for x:

$$\frac{6000x}{6000} = \frac{400}{6000}$$

> Divide both sides by 6000 in order to get x by itself.

$$x = 0.0666 \text{ mL in 1 min}$$
$$x = 0.067 \text{ mL/min}$$

So the rate is 0.067 mL/min.

>>

>>

STAGE 2 CALCULATE FLOW RATE IN ML/H

Formula method

$$\text{Rate (mL/h)} = \text{mL/min} \times 60 \text{ min/h}$$

$$= 0.067 \text{ mL/min} \times 60 \text{ min/h}$$

$$= 4.02 \text{ (round down to one}$$
$$\text{decimal place)}$$

$$= 4 \text{ mL/h}$$

So the infusion pump is set at 4 mL/h to deliver the prescribed 4 microg/min.

Proportions method

| If we have: | 0.067 mL = 1 min |
| Then we want: | x mL = 60 min |

> Ensure you put the same units on the same side of the equation (i.e. here both equations have mL on the left side).

Cross-multiply:

0.067 mL = 1 min

x mL = 60 min

> Multiply everything diagonally
> (i.e. 0.067 × 60 = 4.02 and x × 1 = x).

So:

$$x = 4.02$$

$$x = 4 \text{ mL/h}$$

So the infusion pump rate needs to be set at 4 mL/h to deliver 4 microg/min of adrenaline.

🔍 CLINICAL CASE STUDY (MG/MIN)

Antonnie Saville is a previously fit and healthy man requiring an anti-arrhythmic infusion following a cardiac arrest. He is allergic to amiodarone and therefore has been prescribed lignocaine.

The prescriber has ordered the infusion to be set at a rate of 3 mg/min. The infusion was prepared as per the infusion label.

What do you need to do?

Again, there are a few steps required in these sorts of calculations, but it is very similar to the previous worked example. It is important to remember that the 0.9% saline is a 'type' of intravenous fluid, so the '0.9%' part may be ignored in this case.

Now let's follow the two stages to solving mg/min as detailed above.

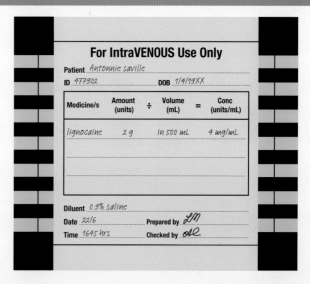

For IntraVENOUS Use Only

Patient _Antonnie saville_
ID _477302_   DOB _1/4/19XX_

Medicine/s	Amount (units)	÷	Volume (mL)	=	Conc (units/mL)
lignocaine	2 g		in 500 mL		4 mg/mL

Diluent _0.9% saline_
Date _22/6_   Prepared by _LM_
Time _1645 hrs_   Checked by _AL_

>>

>>

STAGE 1 CALCULATE RATE IN ML/MIN

Note: 2 g lignocaine = 2000 mg lignocaine

Formula method

$$\text{Rate (mL/min)} = \frac{\text{strength required}}{\text{stock strength}} \times \text{volume}$$

$$= \frac{3 \text{ mg/min}}{2000 \text{ mg}} \times 500 \text{ mL}$$

$$= 0.75 \text{ mL/min}$$

Proportions method

If we have: 2000 mg = 500 mL

Then we   3 mg/min = x mL

want:

| Ensure you put the same units on the same side of the equation (i.e. here both equations have mL on the right side). |

Cross-   2000 mg = 500 mL

multiply: 3 mg/min = x mL

| Multiply everything diagonally (i.e. 2000 × x = 2000x and 500 × 3 = 1500). |

So: 2000x = 1500

Solve for x: $\dfrac{2000x}{2000} = \dfrac{1500}{2000}$

| Divide both sides by 2000 in order to get x by itself. |

$$x = 0.75$$

So the rate is 0.75 mL/min.

STAGE 2 CALCULATE FLOW RATE IN ML/H

Formula method

Rate (mL/h) = mL/min × 60 min/h

$\qquad$ = 0.75 mL/min × 60 min/h

$\qquad$ = 45 mL/h

So the infusion pump is set at 45 mL/h to deliver the prescribed 3 mg/min.

Proportions method

If we have: $\qquad$ 0.75 mL = 1 min

Then we want: $\qquad$ x mL = 60 min

> Ensure you put the same units on same side of the equation (i.e. here both equations have mL on the left side).

Cross-multiply: $\qquad$ 0.75 mL = 1 min

$\qquad\qquad\qquad$ x mL = 60 min

> Multiply everything diagonally (i.e. 0.75 × 60 = 45 and 1 × x = x).

So: $\qquad\qquad\qquad$ x = 45

The infusion pump needs to be set at 45 mL/h to deliver 3 mg/min.

ACTIVITY 9.1

Calculate the expected dose for the client in the following practice questions.

1 Glyceryl trinitrate (GTN) is ordered as a 15 microg/min infusion. The infusion contains 50 mg GTN in 50 mL of 0.9% saline. What rate (mL/h) do you set the infusion pump to?

2 A noradrenaline infusion is ordered for a client at a dose of 12 microg/min. The concentration of the infusion is 4 mg noradrenaline in 50 mL of 0.9% saline. What rate (mL/h) do you set the infusion pump to?

3 A salbutamol infusion is ordered for a client at 15 microg/min. The infusion is prepared as 5 mg salbutamol in 500 mL of 0.9% saline. What rate (mL/h) do you set the infusion pump to?

Infusion calculations – units per body weight per minute (microg/kg/min or mg/kg/min)

As already discussed in previous chapters, some medicines are administered based on the body weight of the client. Because of the potency and danger of some of the medicines used in critical care areas, sometimes medicines are ordered as a dose in microg/kg/min or mg/kg/min.

These calculations are very similar to the microg/min and mg/min infusions we calculated in the previous section; the only difference is that we first need to calculate the total dose for the client based on their body weight – the last two stages of the calculation are exactly as we did in the previous section.

The three key stages to solving microg/kg/min (or mg/kg/min) calculations are shown here.

FORMULA 18 – CALCULATING THE RATE (ML/H) WHEN THE INFUSION IS PRESCRIBED IN UNITS/KG/MIN (MICROG/KG/MIN OR MG/KG/MIN)

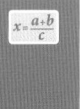

Stage 0 Calculate total amount of medicine needed based on client's body weight (in kg).

Stage 1 Calculate rate in mL/min.

$$\text{Rate (mL/min)} = \frac{\text{strength required}}{\text{stock strength}} \times \text{volume}$$

Stage 2 Calculate flow rate in mL/h.

$$\text{Rate mL/h} = \text{mL/min} \times 60 \text{ min/h}$$

🔍 CASE STUDY (MICROG/KG/MIN)

Caitrine Fisher is a young woman requiring a dobutamine infusion for inotropic support after open-heart surgery. She weighs 71 kg.

The prescriber has ordered the infusion set at a rate of 5 microg/kg/min.

The infusion concentration is as the label.

What do you need to do?

Let's follow the three stages to solving microg/kg/min as detailed above.

STAGE 0 CALCULATE AMOUNT OF MEDICINE REQUIRED BASED ON BODY WEIGHT

If Caitrine weighs 71 kg and you need to give 5 microg dobutamine for every kilogram of her body weight (each minute) then:

71 kg × 5 microg dobutamine = 355 microg dobutamine
each minute is required

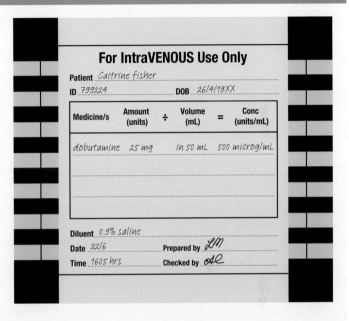

For IntraVENOUS Use Only

Patient _Caitrine fisher_

ID _799224_   DOB _26/4/19XX_

Medicine/s	Amount (units)	÷	Volume (mL)	=	Conc (units/mL)
dobutamine	25 mg	in	50 mL		500 microg/mL

Diluent _0.9% saline_

Date _22/6_   Prepared by _LM_

Time _1605 hrs_   Checked by _AO_

>>

>>

STAGE 1 CALCULATE RATE IN ML/MIN

Note: 25 mg dobutamine = 25 000 microg dobutamine

Formula method

$$\text{Dose (mL/min)} = \frac{\text{strength required}}{\text{stock strength}} \times \text{volume}$$

$$= \frac{355 \text{ microg/min}}{25\,000 \text{ microg}} \times 50 \text{ mL}$$

$$= 0.71 \text{ mL/min}$$

Proportions method

If we have:	25 000 microg = 50 mL
Then we want:	355 microg/min = x mL

Ensure you put the same units on the same side of the equation (i.e. here both equations have mL on the right side).

Cross-multiply: 25 000 microg = 50 mL

355 microg/min = x mL

Multiply everything diagonally (i.e. 25 000 × x = 25 000x and 50 × 355 = 17 750).

So: $25\,000x = 17\,750$

Solve for x: $\dfrac{25\,000x}{25\,000} = \dfrac{17\,750}{25\,000}$

Divide both sides by 25 000 to get x by itself.

$$x = 0.71$$

The rate needs to be 0.71 mL/min.

STAGE 2 CALCULATE FLOW RATE IN ML/H

Formula method

Rate (mL/h) = mL/min × 60 min/h

= 0.71 mL/min × 60 min/h

= 42.6 mL/h

So the infusion pump is set at 42.6 mL/h to deliver the prescribed 5 microg/kg/min for this 71 kg client.

Proportions method

If we have: 0.71 mL = 1 min

Then we want: x mL = 60 min

> Ensure you put the same units on the same side of the equation (i.e. here both equations have mL on the left side).

Cross-multiply: 0.71 mL = 1 min

x mL = 60 min

> Multiply everything diagonally
> (i.e. 0.71 × 60 = 42.6 and 1 × x = x).

So: x = 42.6 mL

So a rate of 42.6 mL/h is needed to deliver the prescribed 5 microg/kg/min for this 71 kg client.

ACTIVITY 9.2

Calculate the expected dose for the client in the following practice questions.

1   Milrinone infusion is ordered for a client (weighing 65 kg) at a dose of 0.75 microg/kg/min. The concentration of the infusion is 10 mg milrinone in 50 mL of 0.9% saline. What rate (mL/h) do you set the infusion pump to?

2   An 83 kg man is prescribed dopamine. The prescribed dose for this medicine is 25 microg/kg/min. What rate (mL/h) do you set the infusion pump to if the infusion has 250 mg dopamine in 50 mL?

3   A woman is ordered an aminophylline infusion to run at a rate of 0.5 mg/kg/h. The client weighs 67 kg and the infusion is made up of 500 mg aminophylline in 50 mL of 0.9% saline. What rate (mL/h) do you set the infusion pump to?

Infusion calculations – bolus infusion doses

Sometimes a client may require a 'bolus' or quick extra dose of a medicine they are receiving via infusion. The most common example of this is a client who is on an analgesic infusion for pain (e.g. morphine) and then requires an extra dose of morphine when they are moved or have their dressings changed.

In order to do this, the infusion concentration must first be known and then the dose needs to be converted to mL (using either proportions method or the standard formula for calculating liquids, as covered in Chapters 5 and 6).

Once the amount of the infusion (in mL) is known, the infusion pump can be programmed to deliver this extra dose of medicine to the client as slowly or quickly as desired (each infusion pump will have a different way of programming the bolus dose). The main piece of information in this instance is the amount of fluid to be given as a bolus dose (the 'volume to be infused'). The rate for this bolus may be 'immediately' (often programmed in as 999 mL/h, which is the quickest that most infusion pumps will run), or the rate (mL/h) may be calculated as shown in the infusions.

SAFETY

THREE STAGES TO ADMINISTERING BOLUS INFUSION DOSES

Stage 1   Calculate the volume of infusion that is required to give a bolus dose.

Stage 2   Program infusion pump to deliver that amount of fluid as the 'volume to be infused'.

Stage 3   Program infusion pump to deliver the dose over the time required as the 'rate' (mL/h).

📋 CLINICAL CASE STUDY (BOLUS INFUSION DOSES)

Alice Janson is a young woman requiring an immediate 5 mg bolus of morphine for a painful procedure. Currently, her morphine is infusing at 4 mL/h and the infusion has been made up as per the concentration label.

How many mL of this infusion is needed to be given as a bolus?

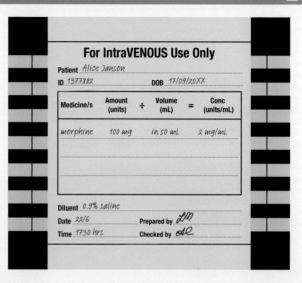

For IntraVENOUS Use Only

Patient _Alice Janson_
ID _1377882_   DOB _17/09/20XX_

Medicine/s	Amount (units)	÷	Volume (mL)	=	Conc (units/mL)
morphine	100 mg		in 50 mL		2 mg/mL

Diluent _0.9% saline_
Date _22/6_   Prepared by _LM_
Time _1730 hrs_   Checked by _AL_

>>

>>

Let's follow the three stages to calculating bolus infusion doses as detailed above.

STAGE 1 CALCULATE VOLUME OF INFUSION REQUIRED BASED ON AMOUNT OF DRUG ORDERED FOR BOLUS DOSE

Formula method

$$\text{Volume required} = \frac{\text{strength required}}{\text{stock strength}} \times \text{volume}$$

$$= \frac{5 \text{ mg}}{100 \text{ mg}} \times 50 \text{ mL}$$

$$= 2.5 \text{ mL}$$

Proportions method

If we have: $100 \text{ mg} = 50 \text{ mL}$

Then we want: $5 \text{ mg} = x \text{ mL}$

> Ensure you put the same units on the same side of the equation (i.e. here both equations have mg on the left side).

Cross-multiply: $100 \text{ mg} = 50 \text{ mL}$

$5 \text{ mg} = x \text{ mL}$

> Multiply everything diagonally (i.e. $100 \times x = 100x$ and $50 \times 5 = 250$).

So: $100x = 250$

Solve for x: $\dfrac{100x}{100} = \dfrac{250}{100}$

> Divide both sides by 100 in order to get x by itself.

$x = 2.5 \text{ mL}$

Volume of infusion for the bolus dose is 2.5 mL.

STAGE 2 PROGRAM INFUSION PUMP TO DELIVER THE CALCULATED VOLUME AS THE 'VOLUME TO BE INFUSED' VIA SECONDARY OR BOLUS PROGRAM

Refer to specific infusion pump instructions for how to do this as each pump will do this slightly differently.

STAGE 3 CALCULATE INFUSION RATE (ML/H) FOR THE BOLUS DOSE

In this case, the bolus is required as quickly as possible, so the secondary infusion rate would be programmed into 999 mL/h

(which is the fastest rate available on most pumps). If a slower rate were required (e.g. if the bolus dose needed to be given over 5 minutes), this would be calculated using the standard rate formula as outlined in Chapter 6 (Infusion calculations).

ACTIVITY 9.3

Calculate the expected dose for the client in the following practice questions.

1   A bolus of 2 mg midazolam is ordered for a client to be delivered over 5 minutes. The infusion has a concentration of 50 mg midazolam in 100 mL 0.9% saline. Calculate the following:
    a   The volume of this infusion you set your infusion pump to deliver as a bolus
    b   The rate (mL/h) you use for this bolus.

2   A bolus of 50 microg of fentanyl is ordered for a client to be delivered over 10 minutes. The infusion has a concentration of 1 mg fentanyl in 100 mL 5% dextrose. Calculate the following:
    a   The volume of this infusion you set your infusion pump to deliver as a bolus
    b   The rate (mL/h) you use for this bolus.

3   Propofol for infusion contains 10 mg of propofol per mL. A client is ordered a 100 mg bolus of this medicine to be given as quickly as possible. Calculate the following:
    a   The volume of this infusion you set your infusion pump to deliver as a bolus
    b   The rate (mL/h) you use for this bolus.

Medicine calculations – liquids and concentrations

The Australian Commission on Safety and Quality in Health Care implemented a program to introduce a consistent method of identifying injectable medicines and fluids and the devices used to deliver them, given that the medicine and diluent cannot be identified by their original packaging once placed in a syringe for administration. These labels require the user to calculate the concentration of the injectable fluid.

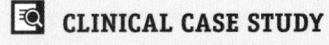

WORKED EXAMPLE 9.5

CLINICAL CASE STUDY

Christopher Nichols is a man who presents with a recent history of cardiac arrest. He has been prescribed an infusion of amiodarone 15 mg per kg over 24 hours diluted up to 500 mL with 5% dextrose. He weighs 79 kg. Amiodarone is available in vials of 150 mg/3 mL.

What do you need to do?

STAGE 0 CALCULATE AMOUNT OF MEDICINE REQUIRED BASED ON BODY WEIGHT

If Christopher weighs 79 kg and you need to give 15 mg amiodarone for every kilogram of his body weight (over 24 hours), then:

79 kg × 15 mg amiodarone = 1185 mg amiodarone over
24 hours is required

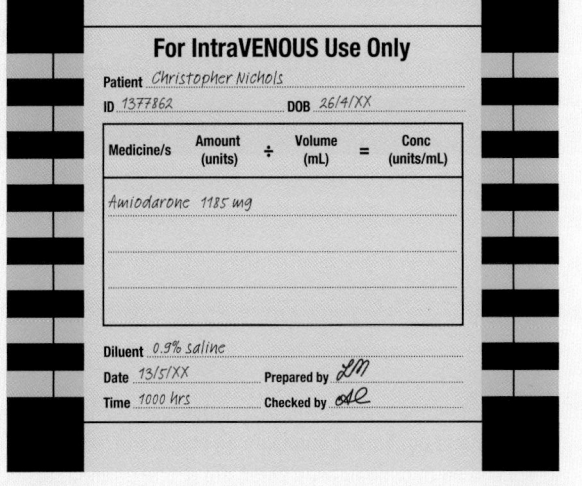

For IntraVENOUS Use Only

Patient _Christopher Nichols_
ID _1377862_   DOB _26/4/XX_

Medicine/s	Amount (units)	÷	Volume (mL)	=	Conc (units/mL)
Amiodarone 1185 mg					

Diluent _0.9% saline_
Date _13/5/XX_   Prepared by _LM_
Time _1000 hrs_   Checked by _AL_

STAGE 1 CALCULATE AMOUNT OF AMIODARONE IN ML

Formula method

$$\text{Dose (mL)} = \frac{\text{strength required}}{\text{stock strength}} \times \text{volume}$$

$$= \frac{1185 \text{ mg}}{150 \text{ mg}} \times 3 \text{ mL}$$

$$= 23.7 \text{ mL}$$

Proportions method

If we have:	150 mg = 3 mL
Then we want:	1185 mg = x mL

Ensure you put the same units on the same side of the equation (i.e. here both equations have mL on the right side).

Cross-multiply: 150 mg = 3 mL
1185 mg = x mL

Multiply everything diagonally (i.e. 150 × x = 150x and 3 × 1185 = 3555).

So: $150x = 3555$

Solve for x: $\dfrac{150x}{150} = \dfrac{3555}{150}$

Divide both sides by 150 to get x by itself.

$$x = 23.74 \text{ mL}$$

We need 23.7 mL of amiodarone 150 mg/3 mL to make up a solution in 5% dextrose 500 mL to give 15 mg/kg over 24 hours.

>>

\>\>

STAGE 2 CALCULATE FLOW RATE IN ML/H

Once we have worked out the amount of amiodarone (150 mg/3 mL) to be diluted with the bag of dextrose (up to 500 mL), we need to calculate the infusion rate over 24 hours.

Formula method

Rate (mL/h) = total volume ÷ 24 h

$$= 500 \text{ mL} \div 24 \text{ h}$$

$$= 20.83 \text{ mL/h}$$

So the infusion pump is set at 20.8 mL/h to deliver the prescribed 15 mg/kg/24 h for this 79 kg client.

If we need a total volume of 500 mL and the bag of dextrose contains 500 mL, then we need to remove 23.7 mL dextrose and discard this before adding the 23.7 mL amiodarone to this bag. This will give us a total volume of 500 mL and contain the required amount of amiodarone.

Proportions method

If we have:	500 mL = 24 h	Ensure you put the same units on the same side of the equation (i.e. here both equations have mL on the left side).
Then we want:	x mL = 1 h	

Cross-multiply:	500 mL = 24 h x mL = 1 h	Multiply everything diagonally (i.e. 500 × 1 = 500 and 24 × x = 24x).

So: $24x = 500$

Solve for x:	$\dfrac{24x}{24} = \dfrac{500}{24}$	Divide both sides by 24 in order to get x by itself.

$$x = 20.833 \text{ mL/h}$$

So a rate of 20.8 mL/h is needed to deliver the prescribed 15 mg/kg/24 h for this 79 kg client.

When completing the infusion label for this scenario, take the total amount of units and divide them by the total volume. This will give a concentration of units/mL.

In this case, the total amount of amiodarone used was 1185 mg in a volume of 500 mL

$$\frac{1185}{500} = 2.37 \text{ mg/mL}$$

Therefore, the concentration for the solution to be infused is 2.37 mg/mL. This is what should be written on the label.

ACTIVITY 9.4

Calculate the expected dose and information for the client in the following practice questions.

1   Kylie is a paediatric client who is commenced on an adrenaline infusion to assist with persistent severe bradycardia. The prescriber has ordered the client to be given adrenaline to commence at a rate of 0.1 microg/kg/min. The child weighs 8.4 kg. Adrenaline is available in a concentration of 1:1000 (0.30 mg/0.30 mL). The infusion is to be made up with 1 mg adrenaline made up to 50 mL with 5% dextrose. Calculate the following:

a   How much adrenaline will be infused per minute?

b   What is the total amount of adrenaline required over a 24-hour period?

c   What is the final concentration in microg/mL?

d   What is the rate (mL/h) you use for this infusion?

e   Complete the following infusion label with the necessary information.

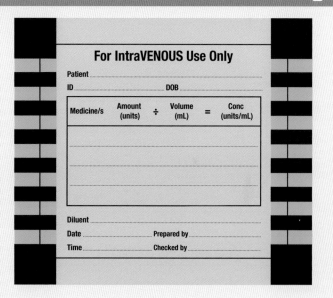

	For IntraVENOUS Use Only	
Patient		
ID	DOB	

Medicine/s	Amount (units) ÷	Volume (mL) =	Conc (units/mL)

Diluent

Date   Prepared by

Time   Checked by

>>

2 Michelle is to be commenced on a dopamine infusion to treat hypotension and low cardiac output. The infusion is to commence at 2 microg/kg/min. The client weighs 82 kg. Dopamine is available in a vial containing 200 mg/5 mL. The infusion needs to contain dopamine 600 mg and is to be made up to 100 mL with sodium chloride.

a How much dopamine will be infused per minute?

b What is the total amount of dopamine required over a 24-hour period?

c What is the rate (mL/h) you will require to administer this infusion?

d Complete the following infusion label with the necessary information.

For IntraVENOUS Use Only

Patient ....

ID .... DOB ....

Medicine/s	Amount (units)	÷	Volume (mL)	=	Conc (units/mL)

Diluent ....

Date .... Prepared by ....

Time .... Checked by ....

10

OTHER SPECIALIST AREAS: AGED CARE, MENTAL HEALTH AND ONCOLOGY

Introduction

Caring for people in specialty areas can be both rewarding and complex. This chapter presents three specialty areas of nursing where there are often bespoke approaches to managing medication. These specialty areas are aged care, mental health and oncology. The three specialty areas are written about together because the knowledge can be synergistic due to the prevalence of potential comorbidities, such as cancer and mental health, in the ageing population. According to the Australian Institute of Health and Welfare (AIHW; 2023a), ageing Australians are living longer and with multiple chronic conditions. The Australian Bureau of Statistics' (ABS) National Health Survey (NHS) estimated that, of the total population of older people (65 years +) in 2017–18, 28 per cent had three or more chronic conditions, while only 20 per cent had none (AIHW, 2023a).

The populations in Australia and New Zealand are ageing steadily and the ABS suggests that up to 27 per cent of the Australian population will be aged 65 years and over by the year 2071, up from 17 per cent in 2022 (ABS, 2023). The ABS also suggests that the proportion of the population aged over 85 will climb from 2.1 per cent in 2022 to as much as 6.4 per cent by 2071.

Simultaneously, the incidence of mental health issues continues to climb. According to the World Health Organization (WHO; 2024), there has been a global increase in mental health disorders, primarily attributed to changes in population dynamics. Despite this increase, the prevalence of mental disorders has remained relatively stable at around 13 per cent (WHO, 2024). This is attributed to the global population expanding at a similar rate during the same period. In 2022, the ABS reported approximately 21 per cent of Australians between the ages of 16 and 85 encountered a mental disorder within the previous 12 months (AIHW, 2023b). In New Zealand, there was a notable rise in the percentage of individuals experiencing low mental wellbeing, from 22 per cent in 2018 to 28 per cent in 2021 (Stats NZ Tatauranga Aotearoa, 2022).

There have also been increases in the number of cases within the field of oncology, the clinical specialty concerned with managing cancer. According to the AIHW (2021), cancer accounts for 18 per cent of the total burden of ill health in Australia. In 2021, the AIHW estimated that 151 000 new cases of cancer (excluding basal cell carcinoma and squamous cell carcinoma) would be diagnosed in Australia, with this number estimated to increase to 185 000 new cases per year by 2031.

Given the projections of an increasing aged population and continuing growth in the areas of mental health and oncology, it is likely that all healthcare professionals will encounter or work with clients in each of these areas at some stage.

Although aged care, oncology and mental health are specialty areas in their own right, there are some core similarities, including the considerations of safety, polypharmacy and therapeutic indexes. Some unique approaches to dosage calculations will also be highlighted in this chapter through these specialist areas.

Considerations common to these specialist areas

Safety

Healthcare professionals may work with ageing, oncology and/or mental health clients in community settings, hospital environments or specialist care facilities. Different locations will have different systems and procedures for managing and administering medicines safely. However, all of these must comply with relevant national and state/territory legislation pertaining to the use of medicines. This resource does not detail these guidelines/laws, as these can be accessed independently.

The '10 steps for safe use of a medication chart' are essential to all areas of nursing.

Polypharmacy

Polypharmacy (the concurrent use of five or more medicines at the same time) can occur with any medicine user. These medicines may be prescribed, complementary (herbal) or 'over the counter' (OTC). The main risks of polypharmacy include drug interactions, adverse drug reactions, unnecessary costs (such as buying two different brands of paracetamol) and an increased risk of confusion and sedation (increasing the risk of falls). The risk of drug interactions or adverse effects increases with each additional medicine.

However, the incidence of polypharmacy may be reduced if a client has a good relationship with their primary care provider and local pharmacist. Regular medicine reviews and clear communication with all members of the healthcare team (including the client) are vital components in managing the risks associated with a client's polypharmacy. The National Safety and Quality Health Service Standards provided by the Australian Commission on Safety and Quality in Healthcare feature medication reviews (Action 4.10) as a requirement of continuity of medication management. A prescriber should consider existing treatments when prescribing new medications or when changing or ceasing medications, by reflecting on evidence-based best practice and a patient's clinical needs. Medication reviews can be informal, multidisciplinary or formal. Home medicines reviews (HMR) and residential medication management reviews (RMMR), for clients in residential aged care, are conducted by approved pharmacists in conjunction with a general practitioner (GP), and can be funded by Medicare every two years.

Mental health conditions often require the use of multiple medications for management, and cancer treatment or 'cancer control' encompasses all means of managing cancer, including radiation, chemotherapy and medications. Treatment involves the use of various medicines in numerous dose forms. These medicines are used for both symptom control (e.g. to control pain or nausea) and in the treatment of the cancer itself. An example of protocols can be found at the Cancer Institute NSW eviQ website (https://www.eviq.org.au), where clinicians can create a login and view the current protocols recommended for various cancers.

The cumulative effects of lifestyle, genetic factors and comorbidities mean that as people get older, there is a higher incidence of disease. Because of this, older people are often required to take more than one medicine to manage their medical conditions. According to the Australian Commission on Safety and Quality in Healthcare (2023), while 40 per cent of people aged over 75 are dispensed five or more medications, approximately two-thirds of this age group take five or more medicines when we include OTC and complementary medicines.

Dementia patients often have complex behaviours that require multidisciplinary and pharmaceutical management. Dementia Australia (2023) strictly advocates for the avoidance of medications unless they are absolutely necessary. On its website, Dementia Australia explores common types of drugs that are often co-prescribed for treatment of symptoms, including those shown in Table 10.1.

TABLE 10.1 Drugs commonly co-prescribed for treatment of dementia symptoms

Symptom	Class	Example
Agitation, aggression and psychotic symptoms	Antipsychotics	Quetiapine
Depression	Antidepressants	Sertraline
Anxiety	Benzodiazepines	Oxazepam
Sleep disturbance	Hypnotics	Zopiclone
Behavioural symptoms (drive, mood, confidence)	Cholinesterase inhibitors	Donepezil

Some more examples of polypharmacy are given in Table 10.2.

TABLE 10.2 Examples of polypharmacy

Polypharmacy	Clinical example
Some clients use medicine that they have no need for.	Client may continue to take/be given an antibiotic for an infection that has long ago resolved.
Some clients use medicines that interact with each other or that are contraindicated.	Client purchases St John's wort for depression from the health food shop, unaware that it interacts with their warfarin. This could cause catastrophic haemorrhage and death.
Some clients take an incorrect dose of the medicine.	Some clients may incorrectly calculate how many tablets to take. Others may halve the prescribed dose in order to make the prescription last longer and reduce the cost of expensive medicines. This is dangerous as the client will get ineffective symptom control and may place their life at risk.
There may be lower rates of adherence to a medicine regimen.	As the number of medicines to be taken increases, a client may forget to take some of the medicines or may refuse to take them all – based on the fact that there are too many.
Clients may confuse the names of medicines and inadvertently take two doses of the same medicine.	Often, clients who take paracetamol refer to it by the trade name (e.g. 'Panadol'). If they are also given another trade brand of paracetamol (e.g. 'Dymadon'), they may take both medicines concurrently, unaware that they are the same. This could lead to overdose and toxicity.
Medicine may be prescribed to manage the adverse effects of other important drugs.	Clients on a diuretic for heart failure lose potassium when they urinate more frequently. In this case, they may need to take a potassium supplement with the diuretic to balance this loss.
Clients may actually require numerous medicines to manage their health condition.	Often, a client may require medicine to treat numerous symptoms or medical conditions (e.g. dementia, schizophrenia). Sometimes these medicines interact or pose a risk to the client, and the benefit of these medicines needs to be compared with the risk of a client *not* taking them.

All health professionals should be alert to the dangers of polypharmacy. Medicines should be reviewed to ensure they are still indicated and safe for the client before dosage calculations are performed.

Therapeutic indexes

All medicines have a therapeutic range – the range of concentration of a medicine required to achieve the desired therapeutic effect without causing toxicity (see Figure 10.1). Some medicines have very narrow therapeutic indexes, with the minimum effective concentration (mec) often being quite close to the maximum safe dose. This creates a very narrow therapeutic window (or index) between the effective dose and the toxic dose, as can be seen in Figure 10.2. Notice the difference between these graphs. In Figure 10.1, you can see a relatively wide therapeutic index (as seen in many commonly used medicines). In Figure 10.2, however, you can see a much narrower window between the minimum effective concentration and the toxic range (maximum effective concentration). Too small a dose will be ineffective, whereas too much could be life-threatening. These medicines require careful calculation of dosage to minimise risks to clients, while ensuring an effective dose is given.

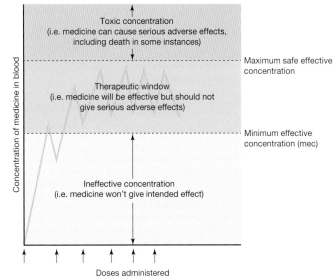

FIGURE 10.1 Graph showing a drug with a wide therapeutic index

FIGURE 10.2 Graph showing a drug with a very narrow therapeutic index

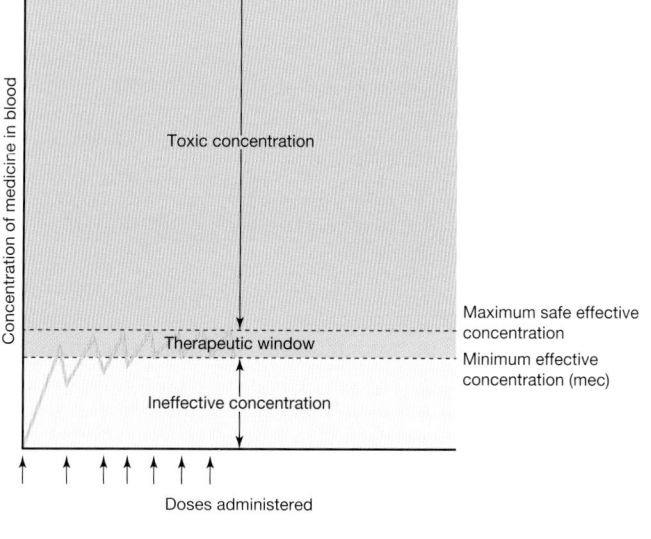

TABLE 10.3 Examples of medications with narrow therapeutic indexes

Medication example	Comment
Lithium	Subtherapeutic risks can include unsuccessful prophylaxis and treatment of mania. Toxic concentrations may include ECG changes, diarrhoea, vomiting, anorexia, abdominal discomfort, polyuria, muscle weakness, ataxia, lethargy, lack of coordination, tinnitus, blurred vision, tremor, muscle twitching, agitation, psychosis, seizure and coma. Plasma lithium concentrations should be checked frequently.
High dose methotrexate	Subtherapeutic risks may include ineffective treatment of cancers such as acute leukaemias. Toxic concentrations cause adverse effects and are generally dose related, including acute and chronic liver toxicity, renal failure, pneumonitis, ulcerative stomatitis, nausea, vomiting, stomach pain, diarrhoea, anorexia and bone marrow depression. MTX monitoring is required.
Warfarin	Subtherapeutic risks include increased risk of clotting. Toxic concentrations substantially increase the risk of bleeding and haemorrhage. INR monitoring is required.

Table 10.3 provides examples of medications used within the three different fields discussed in this chapter that have narrow therapeutic indexes.

Administration of oral dose forms

Oral medications

Many medicines administered in aged care, mental health care and oncology are in forms such as tablets, capsules, wafers, lozenges, liquids, drops and syrups. In most circumstances, they have to be absorbed through the stomach or small intestine to enter the bloodstream. However, based on their action of absorption, there must be careful consideration taken for the correct administration to allow for absorption and/or prevent risk of adverse events due to incorrect administration.

Cutting and crushing tablets

Some clients may often have medical conditions and/or altered cognition that impairs their ability to swallow oral medicines safely. Sometimes a client may be able to swallow a liquid or crushed medicine but is unable to swallow a full tablet or capsule. In this instance, it may be appropriate to either split the tablet or crush the medicine to facilitate oral administration. However, this is not always a safe practice and may not be allowed in some situations and clinical agencies.

Tablets may be scored (Figure 10.3) or unscored (Figure 10.4). A scored tablet has a line etched into the surface of the tablet, making it easier to break in half. An unscored tablet is harder to break in half and is sometimes left unscored to illustrate that it should not be broken at all.

FIGURE 10.3 Scored tablet

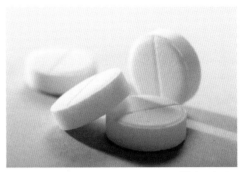

iStock.com/sandsun

FIGURE 10.4 Unscored tablet

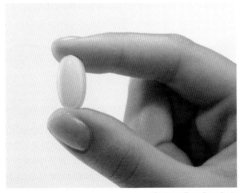

iStock.com/FreezeFrameStudio

Scored tablets may be split into halves or quarters. This enables the client to swallow it more easily; it may also allow a correct dose to be administered. Tablets should usually only be split into halves, as the risk of inaccurate doses increases as a tablet is broken down to quarters. If a tablet is to be split, it is best to use a clean and dry tablet cutter (Figure 10.5) to ensure it is cut evenly. Tablet cutters should be cleaned between clients to reduce the risk of allergy or inadvertent administration of a medicine from one client to the next.

FIGURE 10.5 Tablet splitter

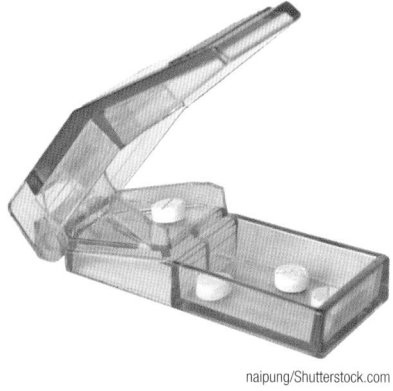

naipung/Shutterstock.com

Split or crushed tablets (or the powder from inside capsules) may be mixed with a small amount of jam or food (Figure 10.6) if this is accepted by the clinical agency and is appropriate for a client (e.g. they may have swallowing difficulties). This may help a client to swallow the medicine if the size of the tablet/ capsule is too big.

FIGURE 10.6 Powdered medicine on jam

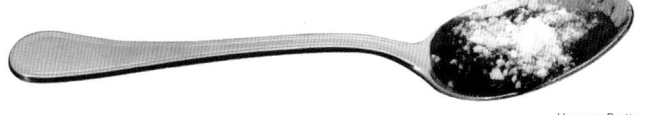

Vanessa Brotto

When an older or palliative care client requires an oral medicine but cannot swallow safely, the drug may need to be administered in another form. This could be parenterally (injection) or rectally, to reduce the risk of choking and aspiration. If a drug cannot be given outside the oral route, the client may need an 'enteral tube', also called a 'feeding tube'. These tubes may be temporary (commonly seen as nasogastric or orogastric tubes) or more permanent (gastronomy or percutaneous gastronomy tubes [PEGs]). These tubes can be used for fluid and feeding, and for administering medicines. The risk with administering medicines into these tubes via syringe is that they may become blocked by the little fragments of tablets. For this reason, it is best to use liquid preparations or to crush tablets/capsule pellets into a fine powder (only if appropriate for that medicine). This is usually done with a pill crusher, a 'mortar and pestle' (Figure 10.7) or using two spoons (Figure 10.8).

The resulting powder is then carefully mixed with water, drawn up in a large syringe and administered into the enteral tube (gradually, without being forced), which is then flushed well with water to prevent it blocking the tube (Figure 10.9).

FIGURE 10.7 Mortar and pestle

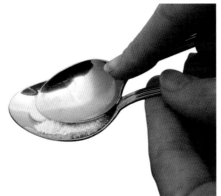

SARANS/Shutterstock.com

FIGURE 10.8 Crushing a tablet using two spoons

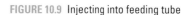

Vanessa Brotto

FIGURE 10.9 Injecting into feeding tube

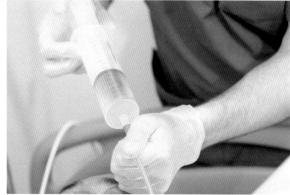

Yuriy Klochan/123RF.com

Tablets with special coatings

Some tablets or pellets from capsules cannot be crushed and they are coated in a special release coating (Figure 10.10). A sustained-release (SR) preparation is one example. Sustained-release tablets are designed to break down slowly in the gastrointestinal tract, releasing a small amount of medicine at intervals so that the medicine may last for up to 24 hours. If these preparations were crushed or chewed, potentially all of the medicine could be released at once, leading to an overdose. Another type of special coating is the enteric coating (EC). This is used to protect the medicine from the harmful acid of the stomach, which may neutralise and destroy more-alkaline drugs. Enteric-coated medicines need the enteric coating to provide a type of armour against the stomach acids until they reach the alkaline small intestine, where they can be safely absorbed. If enteric-coated tablets are broken or chewed, the drug may be totally destroyed in the acidic stomach, leading to no drug being absorbed at all.

FIGURE 10.10 Enteric-coated and sustained-release tablets and capsules

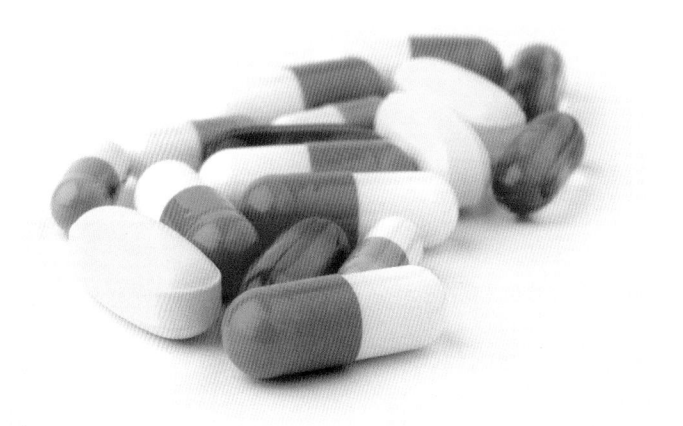

Digieva/Shutterstock.com

Wafers

In the specialty areas of mental health, aged care and oncology, medications may more frequently be in wafer form as well as tablet form (Figure 10.11) and via intramuscular injection (discussed in the next section). The wafer preparations are used when clients are unable to swallow tablets, where it is uncertain if the client will comply with swallowing a tablet or when rapid absorption is required. The wafers are placed on or under the tongue and usually dissolve within seconds.

FIGURE 10.11 Tablet and wafer

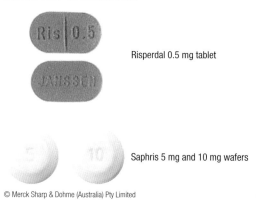

Risperdal 0.5 mg tablet

Saphris 5 mg and 10 mg wafers

© Merck Sharp & Dohme (Australia) Pty Limited

TABLE 10.4 Medications in wafer form

Medication example	Use
desmopressin (Minirin Melt)	primary nocturnal enuresis and cranial diabetes insipidus
ondansetron (Zofran)	control of nausea experienced during chemotherapy
asenapine (Saphris)	schizophrenia or bipolar I disorder (acute mania or maintenance)

Intramuscular injections

Intramuscular injections are a technique of medication delivery that injects a medication deep into the body of a muscle where the medication is generally quickly absorbed into the bloodstream.

Intramuscular injections used in mental health and aged care may be of a medicine in a usual 'for injection' preparation (intermediate-acting) or they may be a 'long acting injectable antipsychotic medication', also known as a 'depot injection'. In a depot injection, the medicine is often suspended in oil, which means that release and absorption takes a long time (over a number of weeks); hence, these formulations are used as longer-term treatment options. Many antipsychotic medications are formulated as depot preparations, so they can be administered once every two to four weeks rather than given daily in tablet form. Antipsychotics can be used in the treatment of mental health conditions and dementia.

In oncology, chemotherapy is less commonly given via intramuscular route. However, medication can be given via this route because it allows for a slower absorption of a chemotherapy medication than by the intravenous route. The Cancer Institute NSW website eviQ provides the instructions for the clinical procedure (administration of anti-cancer drugs – intramuscular and subcutaneous).

Body surface area

In aged care and mental health, complexities of dosing can be affected by extremes of patient size, such as anorexia or morbid obesity. According to Stefani, Singer and Roberts (2019), 'at extremes of body mass, the estimated glomerular filtration rate can under- or overestimate kidney function. It may need to be adjusted for body surface area (BSA), particularly for drugs with a narrow therapeutic range or requiring a minimum concentration to be effective'. However, BSA is more commonly used in paediatrics and oncology.

Chapter 7 described the BSA method as used in paediatrics. Some chemotherapy agents also have doses calculated using this method. The use of BSA in calculating doses in oncology is not without debate and can be problematic. The American Society of Clinical Oncology recommends that the client's actual weight be used, rather than calculating their 'ideal body weight' (Lyman & Griggs, 2012).

Chapter 7 explained the BSA calculation using the Mosteller formula, also referred to as the Mosteller equation (Formula 16), which is one of the four accepted equations used to estimate BSA. The other equations that may be used for this purpose include the DuBois and DuBois formula (referred to as the Du Bois formula or equation and shown in Formula 19), the Gehan and George formula (Formula 20) and the Haycock, Schwartz and Wisotsky formula (referred to as the Haycock formula or equation and shown in Formula 21). Each of these equations will give a slightly different result and so it is important that clinicians use a standardised approach; the Mosteller formula is often utilised because of its ease of use. However, the choice of equation is often made by the prescriber and/or the health agency policies. Many clinicians now use online calculators or smartphone applications to perform these calculations, but they must ensure they are using a consistent formula even when using an online calculator. eviQ includes a BSA calculator, whereby the user can select between the Mosteller or the Du Bois formula.

According to Cancer Council Australia (2023), the Mosteller and Du Bois formulae are the most commonly used formulae. In chemotherapy doses, the nomograms are not often used, as the equations calculate the BSA more accurately. Chemotherapy has such a narrow therapeutic index that its high-risk profile demands doses are calculated as accurately as possible.

Clinical case studies

CLINICAL CASE STUDY: AGED CARE

Mrs Dorothy Tallana is an 86-year-old resident in a long-term aged care facility. She has a past history of asthma and recurrent persistent atrial fibrillation. She was recently diagnosed with cellulitis of her leg and a urinary tract infection, requiring antibiotics and analgesia. Mrs Tallana can swallow tablets, but they make her gag so she prefers them crushed up in jam. She takes her salbutamol in her own private living space and is independent at switching the machine on and off once the measured medication is added to the nebuliser mask by the nurse.

It is now 0800 hrs on 2 April. Refer to Mrs Tallana's medication chart and work through the '10 steps for safe use of a medication chart'.

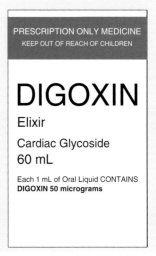

>>

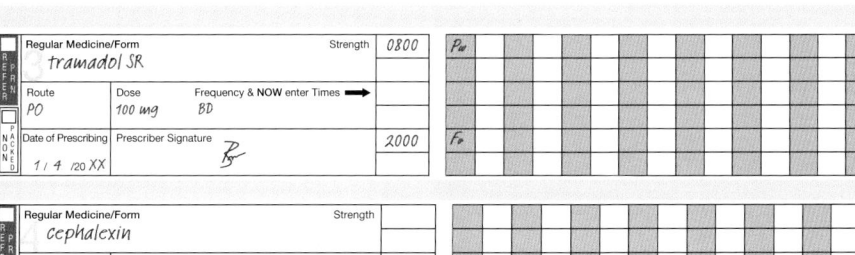

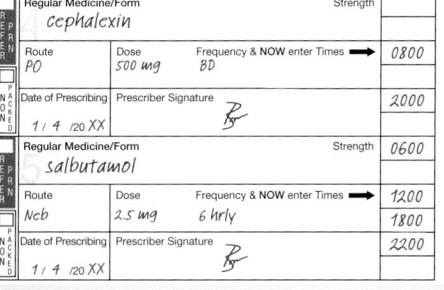

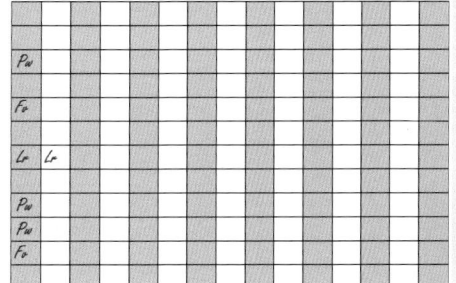

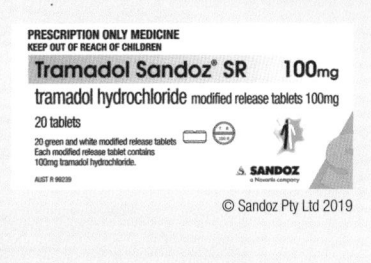

© Sandoz Pty Ltd 2019

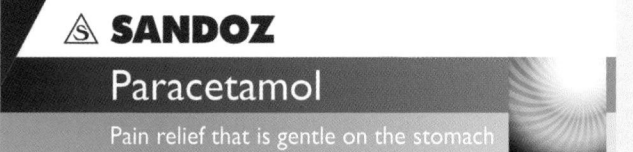

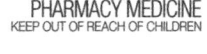

PHARMACY MEDICINE
KEEP OUT OF REACH OF CHILDREN

△ **SANDOZ**

Paracetamol

Pain relief that is gentle on the stomach

Each tablet contains paracetamol 500mg

100 tablets

AUST R 211458

© Sandoz Pty Ltd 2019

PRESCRIPTION ONLY MEDICINE
KEEP OUT OF REACH OF CHILDREN

Salbutamol inhalation ampoules 5 mg/2.5 mL

30 ampoules

Each ampoule with 2.5 mL contains salbutamol
sulphate equivalent to salbutamol 5 mg

In order to calculate what medicine doses are now due, let's review the '10 steps for safe use of a medication chart' as outlined in previous chapters.

SAFETY

10 STEPS FOR SAFE USE OF A MEDICATION CHART

Step 1 Scan medication chart to ensure the prescription(s) are legal and are able to be used.

Step 2 Check which medicines are due/available to administer now.

Step 3 Check for any interactions or contraindications. If medicines have a risk of serious adverse effects, then ensure you are able to monitor/manage these safely.

Step 4 Check that the dosage and route are appropriate for the client's condition.

Step 5 Assess the client to see if the medicine(s) are suitable for them at this time. Ensure no allergies or contraindications to this medicine.

Step 6 Think about this dose – is it logical (e.g. you would not expect to give more than a couple of tablets or a few mL out of a bottle)?

Step 7 Convert all measurements to the same units and then perform dosage calculations using either the formula or the proportions method. This ensures the correct amount of medicine is given.

Step 8 Administer the medicine following the '7 rights', ensuring the client understands and consents to this.

Step 9 Sign/document the medicine as administered on the appropriate charts.

Step 10 Assess the client for any adverse effects.

So let's now work through these steps and calculate the doses.

>>

>>

WORKED EXAMPLE – ANSWERS

Step 1	✓	All prescriptions on this medicine chart are complete and meet legal requirements.
Step 2	✓	All the medicines on this chart are due now at 0800 hrs.
Step 3	✓	No significant interactions/precautions are noted.
Step 4	✓	Dosage and routes are appropriate for the older client.
Step 5	✓	The client has no allergies and has been assessed as being in a stable condition for these medicines.
Step 6	→	Let's work out these dose calculations as shown below …

DIGOXIN

Formula method

$$\text{Dose} = \frac{\text{strength required}}{\text{stock strength}} \times \text{volume}$$

$$\text{Dose} = \frac{125 \text{ microg}}{50 \text{ microg}} \times 1 \text{ mL} \quad \boxed{(125 \div 50, \text{ then} \times 1)}$$

Dose = 2.5 mL digoxin to be administered

Proportions method

If we have: 50 microg = 1 mL
Then we want: 125 microg = x mL

> Ensure you put the same units on the same side of the equation (i.e. here both equations have microg on the left side).

Cross-multiply:

50 microg = 1 mL
125 microg = x mL

> Multiply everything diagonally (i.e. 50 × x = 50x and 125 × 1 = 125).

So: $50x = 125$

Solve for x: $\dfrac{50x}{50} = \dfrac{125}{50}$

> Divide both sides by 50 in order to get x by itself.

$x = 2.5$ mL digoxin

Administer…

Shake the bottle to evenly distribute medicine in the liquid and then draw up 2.5 mL of digoxin in a syringe to administer directly into the client's mouth with the syringe.

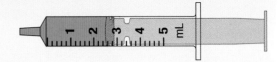

PARACETAMOL

Convert to smaller units; i.e. 1 g = 1000 mg

Formula method

$$\text{Dose} = \frac{\text{strength required}}{\text{stock strength}} \times \text{volume}$$

Ensure strength required and stock strength are in the same units.
(1000 ÷ 500, then × 1)

$$\text{Dose} = \frac{1000 \text{ mg}}{500 \text{ mg}} \times 1 \text{ tablet}$$

Dose = 2 tablets of paracetamol

Proportions method

| Convert to smaller units | 1 g = 1000 mg | Ensure you are dealing with the same units for what you have and what you want. |

| If we have: | 500 mg = 1 tablet | Ensure you put the same units on the same side of the equation (i.e. here both equations have mg on the left side). |
| Then we want: | 1000 mg = x tablets | |

| Cross-multiply: | 500 mg = 1 tablet | Multiply everything diagonally (i.e. 500 × x = 500x and 1000 × 1 = 1000). |
| | 1000 mg = x tablets | |

So: $500x = 1000$

| Solve for x: | $\dfrac{500x}{500} = \dfrac{1000}{500}$ | Divide both sides by 500 in order to get x by itself. |

$x = 2$ tablets of paracetamol

>>

Administer…

Two paracetamol tablets may be split/crushed to make it easier for the client to take the medicine.

TRAMADOL SR

Formula method

$$Dose = \frac{\text{strength required}}{\text{stock strength}} \times \text{volume}$$

$$Dose = \frac{100 \text{ mg}}{100 \text{ mg}} \times 1 \text{ tablet}$$

$(100 \div 100, \text{then} \times 1)$

Dose = 1 tablet of tramadol

Proportions method

| If we have: | 100 mg = 1 tablet |
| Then we want: | 100 mg = x tablets |

Ensure you put the same units on the same side of the equation (i.e. here both equations have mg on the left side).

Cross-multiply:

100 mg = 1 tablet

100 mg = x tablets

Multiply everything diagonally (i.e. $100 \times x = 100x$ and $100 \times 1 = 100$).

So: $100x = 100$

Solve for x:

$$\frac{100x}{100} = \frac{100}{100}$$

Divide both sides by 100 in order to get x by itself.

$x = 1$ tablet of tramadol SR

Administer…

Tramadol SR is a sustained-release tablet that cannot be crushed, split or chewed without risk of serious adverse effects. If the client cannot swallow this tablet, then discuss with the prescriber to change the prescription from the SR preparation.

CEPHALEXIN

Cephalexin is available as 250 mg capsules.

Formula method

$$\text{Dose} = \frac{\text{strength required}}{\text{stock strength}} \times \text{volume}$$

$$\text{Dose} = \frac{500 \text{ mg}}{250 \text{ mg}} \times 1 \text{ capsule}$$

$$\text{Dose} = 2 \text{ capsules cephalexin}$$

(500 ÷ 250, then × 1)

Proportions method

If we have: 250 mg = 1 capsule

Then we want: 500 mg = x capsule

> Ensure you put the same units on the same side of the equation (i.e. here both equations have mg on the left side).

Cross-multiply:

250 mg = 1 capsule

500 mg = x capsules

> Multiply everything diagonally (i.e. $250 \times x = 250x$ and $500 \times 1 = 500$).

So: $250x = 500$

Solve for x: $\dfrac{250x}{250} = \dfrac{500}{250}$

> Divide both sides by 250 in order to get x by itself.

$$x = 2 \text{ capsules of cephalexin}$$

Administer…

These two capsules may be opened and the drug sprinkled into jam to make it easier for the client to take the medicine.

>>

>>

SALBUTAMOL

Formula method

$$\text{Dose} = \frac{\text{strength required}}{\text{stock strength}} \times \text{volume}$$

$$\text{Dose} = \frac{2.5 \text{ mg}}{5 \text{ mg}} \times 2.5 \text{ mL}$$

(2.5 ÷ 5, then × 2.5)

Dose = 1.25 mL of salbutamol

Proportions method

If we have: 5 mg = 2.5 mL
Then we want: 2.5 mg = x mL

| Ensure you put the same units on the same side of the equation (i.e. here both equations have mg on the left side). |

Cross-multiply:

5 mg = 2.5 mL

2.5 mg = x mL

| Multiply everything diagonally (i.e. $5 \times x = 5x$ and $2.5 \times 2.5 = 6.25$). |

So: $5x = 6.25$

Solve for x: $\dfrac{5x}{5} = \dfrac{6.25}{5}$

| Divide both sides by 5 in order to get x by itself. |

$x = 1.25$ mL of salbutamol

Administer...

Shake the bottle to evenly distribute the medicine in the liquid. Draw up the 1.25 mL of salbutamol inhalation solution in a syringe and then place it in the medicine chamber of the nebuliser before turning the unit on and administering it to the client.

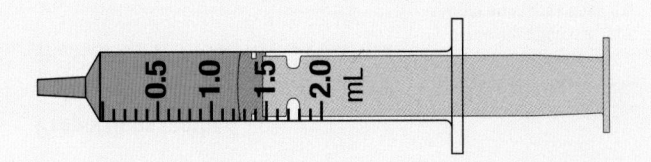

📷 CLINICAL CASE STUDY: AGED CARE

Mr Isidoro Zanbrotto is an 89-year-old man who previously lived at home with his son. He came into hospital following a fall at home two weeks ago, where he was diagnosed with a broken clavicle. Following an Aged Care Assessment, he has just been admitted to Tall Trees Residential Care on the 4 April at 1600 hrs.

He has a past medical history of epilepsy, hypertension, stroke and mild congestive cardiac failure. Following his stroke, Mr Zanbrotto had difficulty swallowing and so a PEG tube was inserted. All fluids, feeds and oral medicines need to be administered via this feeding tube. He also has IV access in his right arm for medications.

1 It is now 0800 hrs on 6 April. Refer to Mr Zanbrotto's medication chart, work through the '10 steps for safe use of a medication chart' and calculate the amount of all medicines to administer.

Resident Name: Isidoro Zanbrotto
D.O.B. 15/2/19XX

Month of April **20** XX

R Refused · A Absent · N Not Available · H Hospital

REGULAR MEDICINES 1 TO 8

Sign in this section for multi-dose administration (eg. multi-dose packs)

Sign in this section for individual medicine administration

Date/Times	1	2	3	4	5	6	7	8	9	10	11	12	13	14	15

Breakfast / Lunch / Dinner / Bed Time

Regular Medicine/Form: atenolol — Strength — 0800
Route: PEG — **Dose:** 25 mg — **Frequency & NOW enter Times:** mane
Date of Prescribing: 4/4/20XX — **Prescriber Signature:** M___

Regular Medicine/Form: phenytoin — Strength — 0800
Route: PEG — **Dose:** 250 mg — **Frequency & NOW enter Times:** mane
Date of Prescribing: 4/4/20XX — **Prescriber Signature:** M___

Regular Medicine/Form: paracetamol — Strength — 0600 / 1200 / 1800 / 2200
Route: PEG — **Dose:** 1 g — **Frequency & NOW enter Times:** QID max. 4 g daily
Date of Prescribing: 4/4/20XX — **Prescriber Signature:** M___

Regular Medicine/Form: frusemide — Strength — 0800 / 1200
Route: IV — **Dose:** 40 mg — **Frequency & NOW enter Times:** BD < mane midi
Date of Prescribing: 4/4/20XX — **Prescriber Signature:** M___

Regular Medicine/Form: digoxin — Strength — 0800
Route: PEG — **Dose:** 125 microg — **Frequency & NOW enter Times:** daily
Date of Prescribing: 4/4/20XX — **Prescriber Signature:** M___

>>

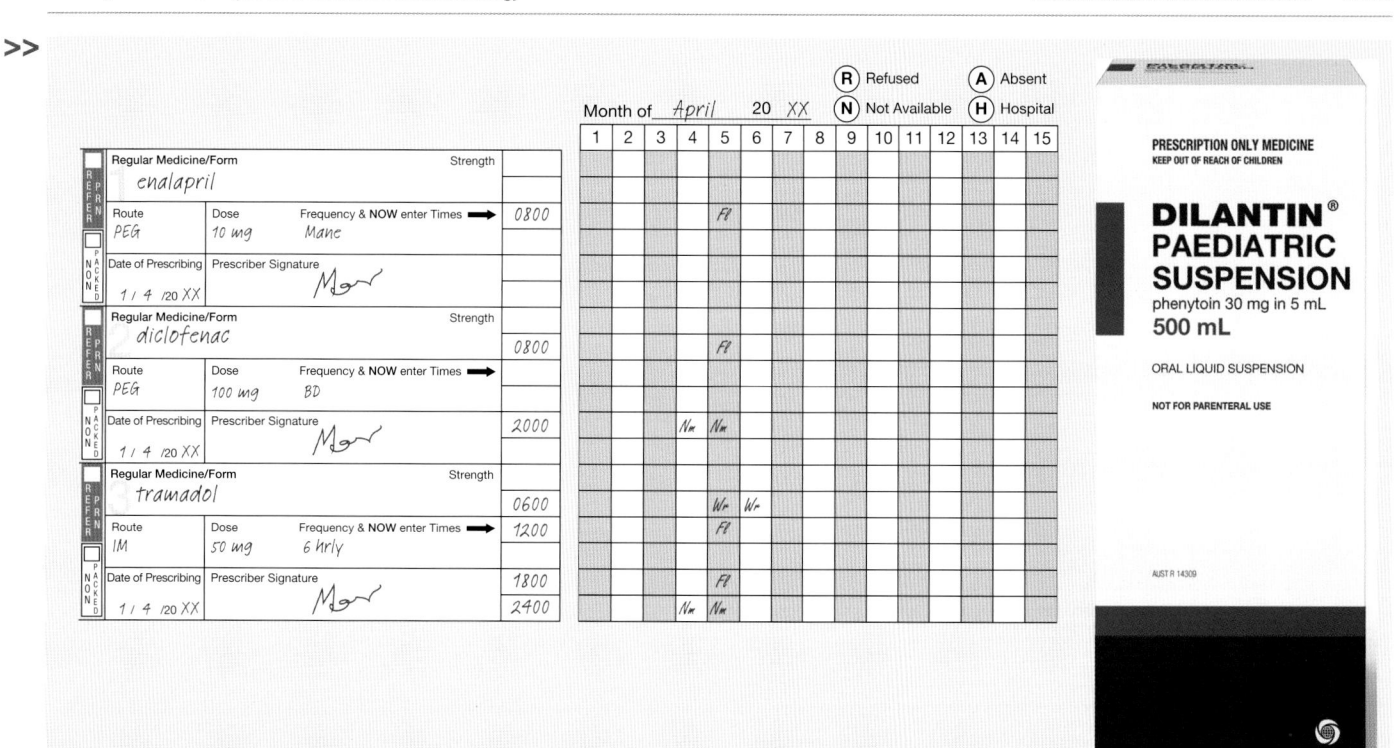

| | R Refused | A Absent |
| | N Not Available | H Hospital |

Month of __April__ 20 __XX__

	1	2	3	4	5	6	7	8	9	10	11	12	13	14	15

Regular Medicine/Form enalapril   Strength

| Route PEG | Dose 10 mg | Frequency & **NOW** enter Times ➡ Mane | 0800 |

Date of Prescribing 1 / 4 /20 XX   Prescriber Signature *Mor*

0800: Fl (col 5)

Regular Medicine/Form diclofenac   Strength

0800

| Route PEG | Dose 100 mg | Frequency & **NOW** enter Times ➡ BD |

2000

0800: Fl (col 5); 2000: Nm (col 4), Nm (col 5)

Regular Medicine/Form tramadol   Strength

0600

| Route IM | Dose 50 mg | Frequency & **NOW** enter Times ➡ 6 hrly |

1200

1800

2400

Date of Prescribing 1 / 4 /20 XX   Prescriber Signature *Mor*

0600: Wr (col 5), Wr (col 6); 1200: Fl (col 5); 1800: Fl (col 5); 2400: Nm (col 4), Nm (col 5)

PRESCRIPTION ONLY MEDICINE
KEEP OUT OF REACH OF CHILDREN

DILANTIN®
PAEDIATRIC
SUSPENSION
phenytoin 30 mg in 5 mL
500 mL

ORAL LIQUID SUSPENSION

NOT FOR PARENTERAL USE

AUST R 14309

VIATRIS

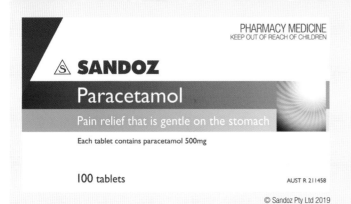

PHARMACY MEDICINE
KEEP OUT OF REACH OF CHILDREN

⚠ SANDOZ

Paracetamol

Pain relief that is gentle on the stomach

Each tablet contains paracetamol 500mg

100 tablets

AUST R 211458

© Sandoz Pty Ltd 2019

PRESCRIPTION ONLY MEDICINE
KEEP OUT OF REACH OF CHILDREN

Lasix ⓓ **20**mg in **2**mL

furosemide (frusemide) injection

Diuretic
Solution for intravenous
or intramuscular injection

AUST R 12404

5 ampoules of **2** mL

SANOFI ⓢ

© Sanofi-Aventis Australia Pty Ltd

PRESCRIPTION ONLY MEDICINE
KEEP OUT OF REACH OF CHILDREN

DIGOXIN

250 micrograms

Digoxin tablets
Each tablet contains DIGOXIN 250 micrograms
100 TABLETS

>>

>>

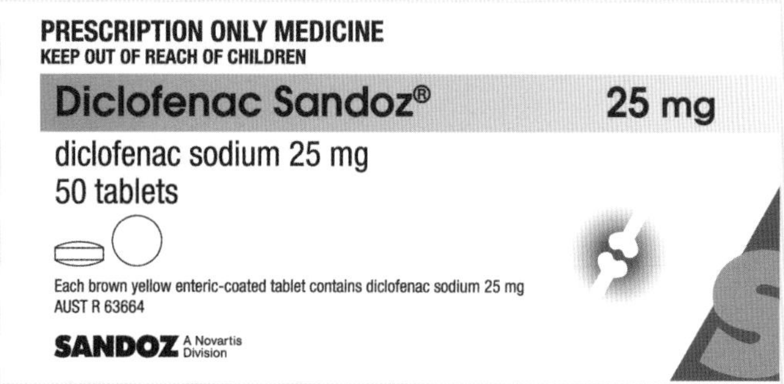

PRESCRIPTION ONLY MEDICINE
KEEP OUT OF REACH OF CHILDREN

Diclofenac Sandoz®   **25 mg**

diclofenac sodium 25 mg
50 tablets

Each brown yellow enteric-coated tablet contains diclofenac sodium 25 mg
AUST R 63664

SANDOZ A Novartis
Division

© Sandoz Pty Ltd 2019

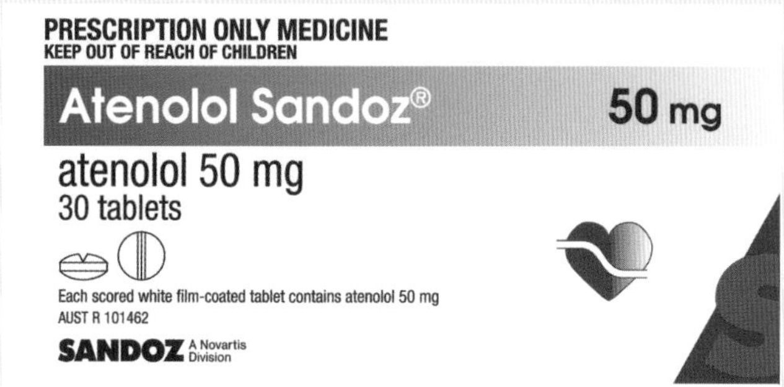

PRESCRIPTION ONLY MEDICINE
KEEP OUT OF REACH OF CHILDREN

Atenolol Sandoz®   **50 mg**

atenolol 50 mg
30 tablets

Each scored white film-coated tablet contains atenolol 50 mg
AUST R 101462

SANDOZ A Novartis
Division

© Sandoz Pty Ltd 2019

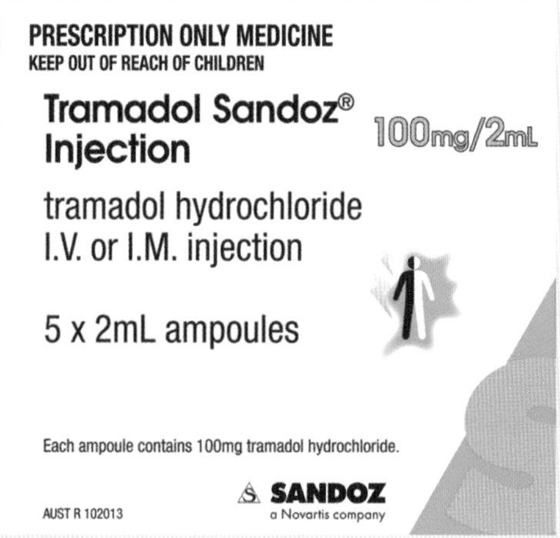

PRESCRIPTION ONLY MEDICINE
KEEP OUT OF REACH OF CHILDREN

Tramadol Sandoz®   100mg/2mL
Injection

tramadol hydrochloride
I.V. or I.M. injection

5 x 2mL ampoules

Each ampoule contains 100mg tramadol hydrochloride.

AUST R 102013   **⚠ SANDOZ**
                       a Novartis company

© Sandoz Pty Ltd 2019

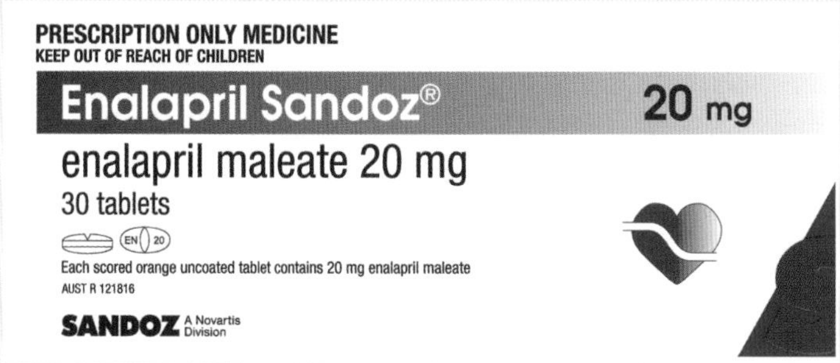

PRESCRIPTION ONLY MEDICINE
KEEP OUT OF REACH OF CHILDREN

Enalapril Sandoz®   **20 mg**

enalapril maleate 20 mg
30 tablets

Each scored orange uncoated tablet contains 20 mg enalapril maleate
AUST R 121816

SANDOZ A Novartis
Division

© Sandoz Pty Ltd 2019

CLINICAL CASE STUDY: MENTAL HEALTH

Campbell Talbot is a 23-year-old man who is currently an inpatient at the mental health unit of a metropolitan hospital. He was admitted with schizophrenia-induced psychosis with paranoid delusions.

It is now 0800 hrs on 25 April. Refer to his medication chart and work through the '10 steps for safe use of a medication chart'.

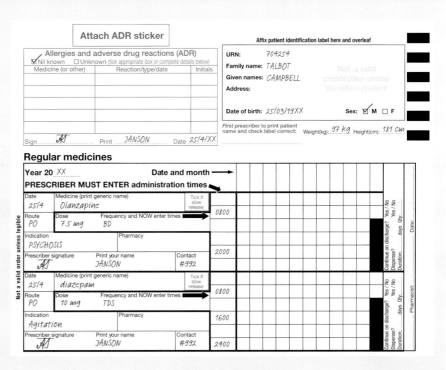

Affix patient identification label here and overleaf

URN:	704254
Family name:	TALBOT
Given names:	CAMPBELL
Address:	

Not a valid prescription unless identifiers present

Date of birth: 25/03/19XX   Sex: ☑ M ☐ F

First prescriber to print patient name and check label correct:

Attach ADR sticker

See front page for details

As required PRN medicines

Year: 20 _XX_

Date 25/4	Medicine (print generic name) chlorpromazine		Date											Continue on discharge? Yes / No	Dispense? Yes / No
Route PO	Dose 100 mg	Hourly frequency 2 Hrly **PRN**	Max PRN dose/24 hrs 500 mg	Time											days Qty:
Indication Agitation		Pharmacy	Dose											Duration:
			Route										
Prescriber signature _AJ_	Print your name JANSON		Contact # 992	Sign										

Date 25/4	Medicine (print generic name) Clopixol (zuclopenthixol)		Date											Continue on discharge? Yes / No	Dispense? Yes / No
Route IM	Dose 150 mg	Hourly frequency Every 3 days **PRN**	Max PRN dose/24 hrs 1 dose in 3 days	Time											days Qty:
Indication Agitation		Pharmacy	Dose											Duration:
			Route										
Prescriber signature _AJ_	Print your name JANSON		Contact # 992	Sign										

Date 25/4	Medicine (print generic name) benztropine		Date											Continue on discharge? Yes / No	Dispense? Yes / No
Route IM	Dose 2 mg	Hourly frequency 12 Hrly **PRN**	Max PRN dose/24 hrs 4 mg	Time											days Qty:
Indication EPS		Pharmacy	Dose											Duration:
			Route										
Prescriber signature _AJ_	Print your name JANSON		Contact # 992	Sign										

Olanzapine Sandoz® ODT 5

olanzapine 5 mg

28 orally disintegrating tablets

Each yellow orally disintegrating tablet contains olanzapine 5 mg

AUST R 179092

SANDOZ A Novartis Division

© Sandoz Pty Ltd 2019

Largactil®

chlorpromazine hydrochloride **25 mg**

Each film-coated tablet contains chlorpromazine hydrochloride 25 mg.

AUST R 51618

100 film-coated tablets

SANOFI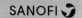

© Sanofi-Aventis Pty Ltd

5 × 1 mL ampoules

Zuclopenthixol ampoules 50 mg/1 mL

Each 1 mL ampoule contains zuclopenthixol acetate equivalent 50 mg (equivalent to zuclopenthixol 45.25 mg) in fractionated coconut oil.

For intramuscular use only

Valpam 5

DIAZEPAM TABLETS

Each tablet contains diazepam 5 mg

50 tablets   AUST R 80811

 SIGMA

© Aspen Australia

>>

>>

PRESCRIPTION ONLY MEDICINE
KEEP OUT OF REACH OF CHILDREN

Benzatropine Injection

benzatropine mesilate 2mg in 2mL injection

Each 2mL contains benzatropine mesilate 2mg, sodium chloride 18mg
in water for injections to 2mL. For intramuscular or intravenous injection.
Use in one patient on one occasion only and discard. Contains no
antimicrobial preservative. This medication may cause drowsiness.
If affected do not drive a vehicle or operate machinery. Avoid alcohol.
Store below 30°C. Protect from light. Do not freeze.

5 x 2mL vials   AUST R 276242 INJ197   **phebra** Ⓟ

© Phebra Pty Ltd

In order to calculate what medicine doses are now available
to administer if required, let's review the '10 steps for safe
use of a medication chart' as outlined in previous chapters.

SAFETY ⚠

10 STEPS FOR SAFE USE OF A MEDICATION CHART

Step 1 Scan medication chart to ensure the prescription(s) are legal and are able to be used.

Step 2 Check which medicines are due/available to administer now.

Step 3 Check for any interactions or contraindications. If medicines have a risk of serious adverse effects, then ensure you are able to monitor/manage these safely.

Step 4 Check that the dosage and route are appropriate for the client's condition.

Step 5 Assess the client to see if the medicine(s) are suitable for them at this time. Ensure no allergies or contraindications to this medicine.

Step 6 Think about this dose – is it logical (e.g. you would not expect to give more than a couple of tablets or a few mL out of a bottle)?

Step 7 Convert all measurements to the same units and then perform dosage calculations using either the formula or the proportions method. This ensures the correct amount of medicine is given.

Step 8 Administer the medicine following the '7 rights', ensuring the client understands and consents to this.

Step 9 Sign/document the medicine as administered on the appropriate charts.

Step 10 Assess the client for any adverse effects.

So let's now work through these steps and calculate the doses.

WORKED EXAMPLE ANSWERS

Step 1	✓	All prescriptions on this medicine chart are complete and meet legal requirements.
Step 2	✓	All the medicines on this chart are available to give now at 0800 hrs (if indicated).
Step 3	✓	No significant interactions/precautions are noted; however, there are a number of antipsychotic drugs and their adverse effects may be serious if used together unnecessarily.
Step 4	✓	Dosage and routes are appropriate for this client.
Step 5	✓	The client has no allergies and has been assessed as being in a stable condition for the 'regular medicines'.
Step 6	→	Let's work out these dose calculations as shown below ...

REGULAR OLANZAPINE

Formula method

$$\text{Dose} = \frac{\text{strength required}}{\text{stock strength}} \times \text{volume}$$

$$\text{Dose} = \frac{7.5 \text{ mg}}{5 \text{ mg}} \times 1 \text{ tablet} \qquad (7.5 \div 5, \text{ then} \times 1)$$

Dose = 1.5 tablets of olanzapine

Proportions method

If we have: 5 mg = 1 tablet
Then we want: 7.5 mg = x tablets

> Ensure you put the same units on the same side of the equation (i.e. here both equations have mg on the left side).

Cross-
multiply:
     5 mg = 1 tablet
     7.5 mg = x tablets

> Multiply everything diagonally (i.e. $5 \times x = 5x$ and $7.5 \times 1 = 7.5$).

So: $5x = 7.5$

Solve for x: $\dfrac{5x}{5} = \dfrac{7.5}{5}$

> Divide both sides by 5 in order to get x by itself.

$x = 1.5$ tablets of olanzapine

>>

Administer…

One and one half tablets of olanzapine are to be given to the client. If the client refuses to take the tablets or if compliance is a problem, the wafer preparation may be preferred.

REGULAR DIAZEPAM

Formula method

$$Dose = \frac{strength\ required}{stock\ strength} \times volume$$

$$Dose = \frac{10\ mg}{5\ mg} \times 1\ tablet \qquad (10 \div 5,\ then \times 1)$$

Dose = 2 tablets of diazepam

Proportions method

If we have: 5 mg = 1 tablet
Then we want: 10 mg = x tablets

> Ensure you put the same units on the same side of the equation (i.e. here both equations have mg on the left side).

Cross-
multiply: 5 mg = 1 tablet

                10 mg = x tablets

> Multiply everything diagonally (i.e. $5 \times x = 5x$ and $10 \times 1 = 10$).

So: $5x = 10$

Solve for x: $\dfrac{5x}{5} = \dfrac{10}{5}$

> Divide both sides by 5 in order to get x by itself.

x = 2 tablets of diazepam

Administer…

Two tablets of diazepam should be administered.

PRN CHLORPROMAZINE

Formula method

$$Dose = \frac{strength\ required}{stock\ strength} \times volume$$

$$Dose = \frac{100\ mg}{25\ mg} \times 1\ tablet \qquad \boxed{(100 \div 25,\ then \times 1)}$$

Dose = 4 tablets of chlorpromazine

Proportions method

If we have:	25 mg = 1 tablet	
Then we want:	100 mg = x tablets	Ensure you put the same units on the same side of the equation (i.e. here both equations have mg on the left side).

Cross-multiply:

25 mg = 1 tablet

100 mg = x tablets

Multiply everything diagonally (i.e. $25 \times x = 25x$ and $100 \times 1 = 100$).

So: $25x = 100$

Solve for x: $\dfrac{25x}{25} = \dfrac{100}{25}$

Divide both sides by 25 in order to get x by itself.

x = 4 tablets of chlorpromazine

Administer…

If chlorpromazine is required, 4 tablets would need to be administered. In this instance, it may be advisable to seek a higher stock strength preparation to reduce the number of tablets this client needs to take (i.e. use the 100 mg strength tablets, if available, rather than the 25 mg tablets).

>>

\>\>

PRN ZUCLOPENTHIXOL

Formula method

$$\text{Dose} = \frac{\text{strength required}}{\text{stock strength}} \times \text{volume}$$

$$\text{Dose} = \frac{150 \text{ mg}}{50 \text{ mg}} \times 1 \text{ mL}$$ (150 ÷ 50, then × 1)

Dose = 3 mL of zuclopenthixol for injection

Proportions method

If we have: 50 mg = 1 mL
Then we want: 150 mg = x mL

> Ensure you put the same units on the same side of the equation (i.e. here both equations have mg on the left side).

Cross-multiply: 50 mg = 1 mL
                              150 mg = x mL

> Multiply everything diagonally (i.e. 50 × x = 50x and 150 × 1 = 150).

So: 50x = 150

Solve for x: $\dfrac{50x}{50} = \dfrac{150}{50}$

> Divide both sides by 50 to get x by itself.

x = 3 mL of zuclopenthixol for injection

Administer...

If zuclopenthixol is required, 3 mL of the drug needs to be administered via intramuscular injection.

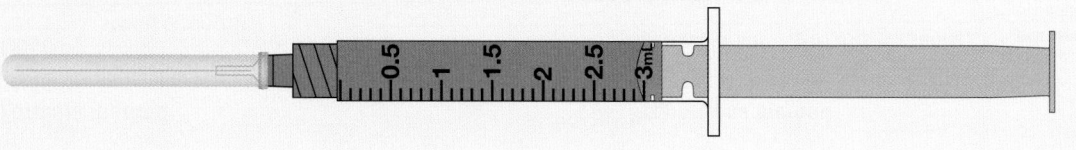

PRN BENZTROPINE

Formula method

$$\text{Dose} = \frac{\text{strength required}}{\text{stock strength}} \times \text{volume}$$

$$\text{Dose} = \frac{2 \text{ mg}}{2 \text{ mg}} \times 2 \text{ mL} \qquad \boxed{(2 \div 2, \text{ then} \times 2)}$$

Dose = 2 mL of benztropine for injection

Proportions method

If we have:	2 mg = 2 mL
Then we want:	2 mg = x mL

Ensure you put the same units on the same side of the equation (i.e. here both equations have mg on the left side).

Cross-multiply:

2 mg = 2 mL

2 mg = x mL

Multiply everything diagonally (i.e. $2 \times x = 2x$ and $2 \times 2 = 4$).

So: $2x = 4$

Solve for x: $\dfrac{2x}{2} = \dfrac{4}{2}$

Divide both sides by 2 to get x by itself.

x = 2 mL of benztropine for injection

Administer…

If benztropine is required, 2 mL of the drug needs to be administered via intramuscular injection.

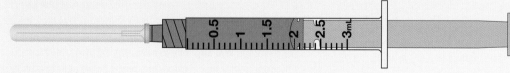

ACTIVITY 10.2

🔍 CLINICAL CASE STUDY: MENTAL HEALTH

Amalie Sienne is a 25-year-old woman who was diagnosed with bipolar disorder three years ago. She was admitted to the inpatient mental health unit when her parents returned from a weekend holiday to find she had spent over $5000 on shoes and was in an agitated state of mania.

Amalie is currently in a manic phase of her illness. It is now 0800 hrs on 25 April 2019.

1 Refer to Amalie's medication chart and work through the '10 steps for safe use of a medication chart'. Calculate the doses for all medicines that are due or available (if required) at this time.

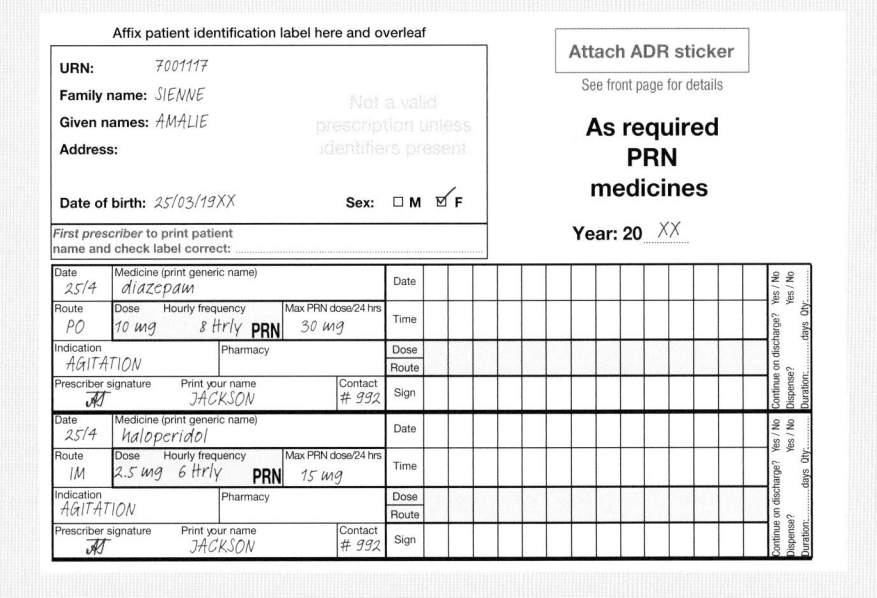

Attach ADR sticker

Allergies and adverse drug reactions (ADR)
☑ Nil known ☐ Unknown (tick appropriate box or complete details below)

Drug (or other)	Reaction/type/date	Initials

Sign _AJ_ Print _JANSON_ Date _25/4/XX_

URN: _7001117_
Family name: _SIENNE_
Given names: _AMALIE_
Address:

Date of birth: _25/03/19XX_ Sex: ☐ M ☑ F

First prescriber to print patient name and check label correct: Weight(kg): _97 kg_ Height(cm): _181 cm_

Regular medicines

Year 20 _XX_ ← Date and month →

PRESCRIBER MUST ENTER administration times

Date 25/4	Medicine (print generic name) _Chlorpromazine_	Tick if slow release	0800	
Route PO	Dose 12.5 mg	Frequency and NOW enter times BD		
Indication BIPOLAR	Pharmacy		2000	
Prescriber signature AJ	Print your name JANSON	Contact #992		
Date 25/4	Medicine (print generic name) _lithium_	Tick if slow release	0800	
Route PO	Dose 500 mg	Frequency and NOW enter times BD		
Indication BIPOLAR	Pharmacy		2000	
Prescriber signature AJ	Print your name JANSON	Contact #992		
Date 25/4	Medicine (print generic name) _diazepam_	Tick if slow release	0600	
Route IV	Dose 5 mg	Frequency and NOW enter times QID	1200	
Indication AGITATION	Pharmacy		1800	
			2400	
Prescriber signature AJ	Print your name JANSON	Contact #992		
Date 25/4	Medicine (print generic name) _temazepam_	Tick if slow release		
Route PO	Dose 20 mg	Frequency and NOW enter times Nocte		
Indication INSOMNIA	Pharmacy		2200	
Prescriber signature AJ	Print your name JANSON	Contact #992		

Not a valid order unless legible

Continue on discharge? Yes / No Dispense? Yes / No Qty ...... days Duration: ...... Date: ...... Pharmacist: ......

>>

>>

PRESCRIPTION ONLY MEDICINE
KEEP OUT OF REACH OF CHILDREN

CHLORPROMAZINE HYDROCHLORIDE

25 mg

Each tablet contains CHLORPROMAZINE
HYDROCHLORIDE 25 mg
100 TABLETS

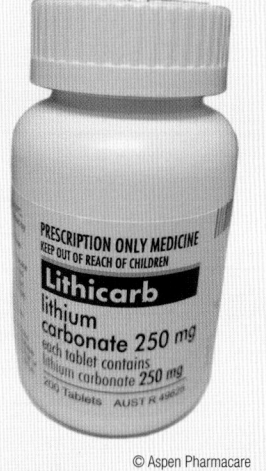

© Aspen Pharmacare

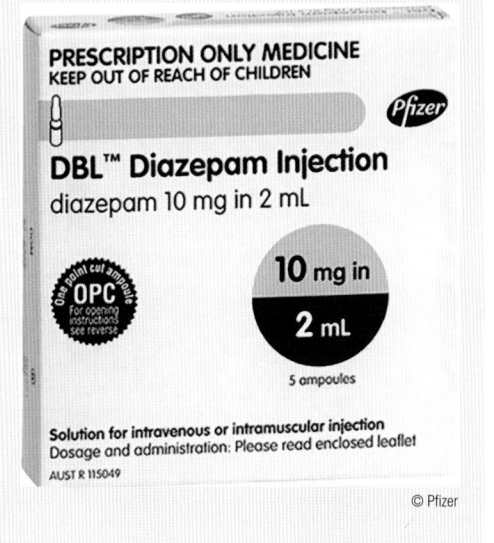

PRESCRIPTION ONLY MEDICINE
KEEP OUT OF REACH OF CHILDREN

Pfizer

DBL™ Diazepam Injection
diazepam 10 mg in 2 mL

OPC
For opening instructions see reverse

10 mg in 2 mL

5 ampoules

Solution for intravenous or intramuscular injection
Dosage and administration: Please read enclosed leaflet

AUST R 115049

© Pfizer

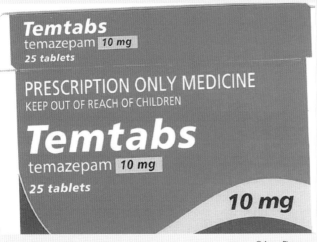

© Aspen Pharmacare

PRESCRIPTION ONLY MEDICINE
KEEP OUT OF REACH OF CHILDREN

Valpam 5

DIAZEPAM TABLETS

Each tablet contains diazepam 5 mg

50 tablets   AUST R 80811

© Aspen Pharmacare

PRESCRIPTION ONLY MEDICINE
KEEP OUT OF REACH OF CHILDREN

10 Ampoules of 1 mL

Serenace Injection

5mg Haloperidol

Each 1 mL Ampoule contains:
HALOPERIDOL 5 mg
INTRAMUSCULAR OR INTRAVENOUS

Excipients: (s)-Lactic acid 0.02 mL/mL
Sodium hydroxide 1.8 mg/mL
Water for injections q.s. 1.0 mL

These ampoules should not be exposed to light

STORE BELOW 30°C.

See enclosed leaflet for directions

In Australia, Consumer Medicine Information is
available from your pharmacist or
www.aspencmi.com.au   AUST R 188367

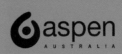

© Aspen Pharmacare

WORKED EXAMPLE 10.3

 CLINICAL CASE STUDY: ONCOLOGY

Mrs Sarah Harris is a 38-year-old woman who is currently a client in the oncology unit of a metropolitan hospital. She was admitted for the treatment of cervical cancer. She weighs 70 kg and is 164 cm tall. She is taking many medicines in this admission to treat her pain and nausea, and to reduce other adverse effects of her treatment. She is now to commence chemotherapy with intravenous cisplatin 40 mg/m².

In order to calculate this dose, we must first calculate Sarah's BSA. This must be done using one of the four approved equations. The equations must be followed exactly and so the proportions method does not apply here. You will note in the following examples that each equation gives a slightly different answer and thus demonstrates the importance of using one standard equation across a health service to keep consistency. Clinicians should familiarise themselves with the preferred equation for where they work. It is not necessary to calculate the BSA using all of the four equations; however, this will be done here to show how to use each formula.

FORMULA 16 – BODY SURFACE AREA (BSA) USING THE MOSTELLER FORMULA

The calculation of BSA using this equation needs to be done using a calculator that has a square root function (see diagram below).

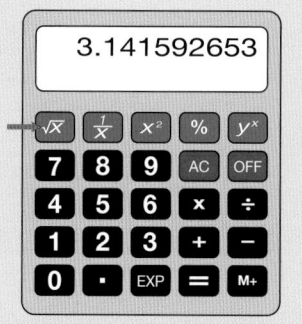

The BSA calculations that are given in this text are obtained by multiplying the height by the weight. This answer is then divided by 3600. Following this, enter the $\sqrt{x}$. This will give the client's BSA in square metres.

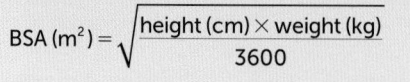

$$\text{BSA (m}^2) = \sqrt{\dfrac{\text{height (cm)} \times \text{weight (kg)}}{3600}}$$

MOSTELLER FORMULA

$$\text{BSA (m}^2) = \sqrt{\frac{\text{height (cm)} \times \text{weight (kg)}}{3600}}$$

$$= \sqrt{\frac{164 \text{ cm} \times 70 \text{ kg}}{3600}}$$

$$= \sqrt{\frac{11\,480}{3600}}$$

$$= \sqrt{3.18888}$$

$$= 1.79 \text{ m}^2$$

The calculation of BSA using this equation needs to be done using a calculator that has an exponential function.

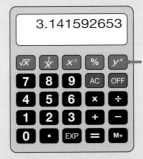

Start by calculating the weight (in kg) to an exponential (also termed as 'to the power of') of 0.425. On the calculator, enter the weight, then press the exponential function key and enter the exponential (i.e. 0.425) and press the equals button to perform the calculation. Then calculate the height (in cm) to an exponential of 0.725. Substitute these values into the equation below and then calculate. This will give the client's BSA in square metres.

$$\text{BSA (m}^2) = 0.007184 \times \text{weight (kg)}^{0.425} \times \text{height (cm)}^{0.725}$$

>>

>>

DU BOIS FORMULA

BSA (m^2) = 0.007184 × weight (kg)$^{0.425}$
           × height (cm)$^{0.725}$

       = 0.007184 × ($70^{0.425}$) × ($164^{0.725}$)

       = 0.007184 × 6.0837 × 40.3424

       = 1.76 m^2

GEHAN AND GEORGE FORMULA

BSA (m^2) = 0.0235 × height (cm)$^{0.42246}$ × weight (kg)$^{0.51456}$

       = 0.0235 × ($164^{0.42246}$) × ($70^{0.51456}$)

       = 0.0235 × 8.6234 × 8.9004

       = 1.80 m^2

FORMULA 20 – BODY SURFACE AREA (BSA) USING THE GEHAN AND GEORGE FORMULA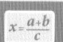

The calculation of BSA using the Gehan and George formula needs to be done using a calculator that has an exponential function. Start by calculating the height (in cm) to an exponential of 0.42246. Then calculate the weight (in kg) to an exponential of 0.51456. Substitute these values into the equation below and then calculate. This will give the client's BSA in square metres.

$$BSA (m^2) = 0.0235 \times height (cm)^{0.42246} \times weight (kg)^{0.51456}$$

FORMULA 21 – BODY SURFACE AREA (BSA) USING THE HAYCOCK FORMULA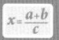

The calculation of BSA using the Haycock formula equation needs to done using a calculator that has an exponential function. Start by calculating the height (in cm) to an exponential of 0.3964. Then calculate the weight (in kg) to an exponential of 0.5378. Substitute these values into the equation below and then calculate. This will give the client's BSA in square metres.

$$BSA (m^2) = 0.024265 \times height (cm)^{0.3964} \times weight (kg)^{0.5378}$$

HAYCOCK EQUATION

$$BSA\ (m^2) = 0.024265 \times height\ (cm)^{0.3964} \times weight\ (kg)^{0.5378}$$
$$= 0.024265 \times (164^{0.3964}) \times (70^{0.5378})$$
$$= 0.024265 \times 7.5502 \times 9.8241$$
$$= 1.80\ m^2$$

CLINICAL CASE STUDY *(CONTINUED)*

Sarah's chemotherapy is intravenous cisplatin 40 mg/m² and from the above calculations we know her BSA is 1.79 m², using the Mosteller equation (note that the prescriber should use the equation chosen as standard by the health agency to ensure a consistent approach to dosing). In order to calculate her dose, we can either modify the formula for dose/kg (Formula 4) or use the proportions method as shown below.

FORMULA 22 – DOSE PER BSA (m²)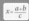

$$Dose = dose/m^2 \times BSA\ in\ m^2$$

Where:
- 'dose/m²' has been prescribed or recommended in a chemotherapy treatment protocol.

Formula method

$$Dose = dose/m^2 \times BSA\ in\ m^2$$
$$= 40 \times 1.79$$
$$= 71.6\ mg\ cisplatin$$

Proportions method

If we have: 40 mg cisplatin = 1 m²

Then we want: x mg = 1.79 m²

> Ensure you put the same units on the same side of the equation (i.e. here both equations have mg on the left side).

Cross-multiply: 40 mg = 1 m²

x mg = 1.79 m²

> Multiply everything diagonally (e.g. 40 × 1.79 = 71.6 and 1 × x = x).

So: $71.6 = 1x$

Solve for x: $\dfrac{71.6}{1} = \dfrac{1x}{1}$

> Divide both sides by 1 in order to get x by itself.

$$x = 71.6\ mg\ cisplatin$$

>>

>>

 CLINICAL CASE STUDY *(CONTINUED)*

Sarah's chemotherapy is intravenous cisplatin 40 mg/m², which has been calculated as being a dose of 71.6 mg cisplatin. What amount will you expect to administer if the following preparation of cisplatin is used?

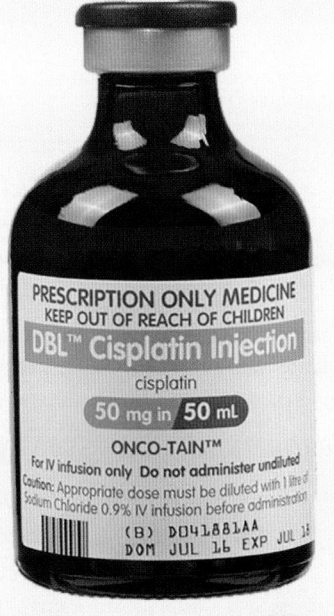

© Pfizer

FORMULA 5 – DOSAGE CALCULATIONS: TABLETS AND LIQUIDS

$$x = \frac{a \cdot b}{c}$$

$$Dose = \frac{strength\ required}{stock\ strength} \times volume$$

Where:

- 'strength required' is the required dose
- 'stock strength' is the concentration of the stock you have ready to administer from
- 'volume' is the amount related to the 'stock strength' (e.g. if you have 5 mg in one tablet, the stock strength is 5 mg and the volume [quantity] is 1 tablet. If you have a liquid of concentration 10 mg/2 mL, the stock strength is 10 mg and the volume is 2 mL).

Formula method

$$\text{Dose} = \frac{\text{strength required}}{\text{stock strength}} \times \text{volume}$$

$$\text{Dose} = \frac{71.6 \text{ mg}}{50 \text{ mg}} \times 50 \text{ mL} \quad \boxed{(71.6 \div 50, \text{ then} \times 50)}$$

Dose = 71.6 mL of cisplatin for injection

Proportions method

If we have: 50 mg cisplatin = 50 mL

Then we want: 71.6 mg = x mL

> Ensure you put the same units on the same side of the equation (i.e. here both equations have mg on the left side).

Cross-multiply:

50 mg = 50 mL

71.6 mg = x mL

> Multiply everything diagonally (i.e. 50 × x = $50x$ and 71.6 × 50 = 3580).

So: $50x = 3580$

Solve for x: $\dfrac{50x}{50} = \dfrac{3580}{50}$

> Divide both sides by 50 in order to get x by itself.

$x = 71.6$ mL cisplatin

>>

>>

 CLINICAL CASE STUDY *(CONTINUED)*

Sarah's intravenous cisplatin is prescribed to be diluted up to 1000 mL of sodium chloride (i.e. 71.6 mL of cisplatin + 928.4 mL of sodium chloride = 1000 mL total volume) and infused over 2 hours via an infusion pump. You now need to calculate the rate (mL/h) that the infusion pump needs to be set at. In order to do this, you can either use the infusion rate formula (as discussed in Chapter 6) or use the proportions method, as shown below.

Formula method

$$\text{Rate (mL/h)} = \frac{\text{total volume of fluid to be infused (mL)}}{\text{time (in hours)}}$$

$$\text{Rate (mL/h)} = \frac{1000 \text{ mL}}{2 \text{ h}}$$

$$\text{Rate (mL/h)} = 500 \text{ mL/h}$$

FORMULA 12 – mL/h (WHEN TIME IS KNOWN IN HOURS)

$$x = \frac{a + b}{c}$$

$$\text{Rate (mL/h)} = \frac{\text{total volume of fluid to be infused (mL)}}{\text{time (in hours)}}$$

Proportions method

If we have:	1000 mL = 2 h	Ensure you put the same units on the same side of the equation (i.e. here both equations have mL on the left side).
Then we want:	x mL = 1 h	

Cross-multiply:	1000 mL = 2 h x mL = 1 h	Multiply everything diagonally (i.e. 1000 × 1 = 1000 and 2 × x = 2x)

So: 1000 = 2x

Solve for x:	$\dfrac{1000}{2} = \dfrac{2x}{2}$	Divide both sides by 2 in order to get x by itself.

$$x = 500 \text{ mL/h}$$

The infusion pump is set at a rate of 500 mL/h.

CLINICAL CASE STUDY: ONCOLOGY

Ms Grace Harris is a 42-year-old woman who has been diagnosed with breast cancer. She weighs 65 kg and is 170 cm tall, and is to have doxorubicin with a dose of 60 mg/m².

1 Calculate her BSA using all of the four different BSA equations.
2 Using your answer to the Mosteller formula, calculate the dose of doxorubicin to be prescribed in mg.
3 What amount will you expect to administer if the following preparation of doxorubicin is used?
4 Doxorubicin is ordered to be infused in 50 mL of normal saline over 15 minutes. What rate do you set the infusion pump to deliver this?

PRESCRIPTION ONLY MEDICINE

KEEP OUT OF REACH OF CHILDREN

DOXORUBICIN HYDROCHLORIDE
50 mg/25 mL

FOR INTRAVENOUS INFUSION ONLY

50 mg/25 mL
Concentrate for Infusion
ONE SINGLE DOSE VIAL

PART 3

SKILLS PRACTICE

PRACTICE QUESTIONS

This chapter has been designed to give you an additional opportunity to practise skills you have gained from other chapters.

Basic mathematics

Basic arithmetic

1	$2 + 6 + 3 + 8 =$	**12**	$72 \times 9 =$
2	$49 + 25 =$	**13**	$1599 \times 8 =$
3	$296 + 91 + 104 + 1 =$	**14**	$4852 \times 45 =$
4	$217 + 896 =$	**15**	$9889 \times 72 =$
5	$12 + 356 + 22 + 33 =$	**16**	$33 \div 3 =$
6	$521 - 86 =$	**17**	$84 \div 6 =$
7	$156 - 69 =$	**18**	$375 \div 5 =$
8	$4589 - 2351 =$	**19**	$1827 \div 29 =$
9	$4892 - 68 =$	**20**	$3906 \div 42 =$
10	$86 - 21 =$		
11	$83 \times 16 =$		

Fractions and decimals

Simplify the following fractions:

21 $\dfrac{8}{24} =$ **28** $\dfrac{23}{6} =$ **35** $\dfrac{2}{5} \times \dfrac{7}{22} =$

22 $\dfrac{25}{1000} =$ **29** $6\dfrac{3}{6} =$ **36** $\dfrac{3}{12} \div \dfrac{2}{5} =$

23 $\dfrac{13}{39} =$ **30** $\dfrac{23}{18} =$ **37** $\dfrac{1}{2} \div \dfrac{9}{11} =$

24 $12\dfrac{4}{8} =$ **31** $\dfrac{1}{6} \times \dfrac{2}{23} =$ **38** $\dfrac{3}{11} \div \dfrac{2}{5} =$

25 $4\dfrac{22}{30} =$ **32** $\dfrac{17}{23} \times \dfrac{5}{9} =$ **39** $\dfrac{6}{8} \div \dfrac{8}{12} =$

26 $\dfrac{27}{5} =$ **33** $\dfrac{3}{8} \times \dfrac{7}{12} =$ **40** $\dfrac{13}{22} \div \dfrac{3}{4} =$

27 $\dfrac{19}{8} =$ **34** $\dfrac{1}{3} \times \dfrac{2}{9} =$

Convert the following fractions to decimals:

41 $\dfrac{43}{50} =$ **42** $\dfrac{22}{25} =$ **43** $\dfrac{13}{50} =$

44 $\dfrac{61}{100} =$ **45** $\dfrac{7}{42} =$

Basic functions with decimals:

46 0.145 + 2.356 =   **56** 8.73 × 710 =

47 0.062 + 0.036 =   **57** 54.65 × 26.8 =

48 0.078 + 0.018 =   **58** 767 × 7.26 =

49 5.698 + 2.359 =   **59** 12.25 × 23.12 =

50 0.081 + 5.200 =   **60** 3.51 × 219 =

51 91.4 − 8.58 =   **61** 2.89 ÷ 1.70 =

52 5.367 − 1.589 =   **62** 45.15 ÷ 5 =

53 10.40 − 2.09 =   **63** 1.26 ÷ 9 =

54 68.40 − 8.08 =   **64** 2.66 ÷ 1.4 =

55 58.63 − 31.89 =   **65** 262.6 ÷ 10.4 =

Conversion

Convert the following:

66 **(a)**   475 mg =   g
   (b)   3750 mL =   L
   (c)   245 microg =   mg
   (d)   750 mg =   g
   (e)   35 g =   mg
   (f)   750 mg =   microg

General questions

1–8. Work out the millilitres to be given for the indicated dose (round the answer off to the nearest tenth of a mL):

Prescriber's order (dose required)	Strength available
1 Erythromycin suspension 120 mg	200 mg/5 mL
2 Erythromycin suspension 333 mg	200 mg/5 mL
3 Erythromycin suspension 200 mg	400 mg/5 mL
4 Erythromycin suspension 250 mg	400 mg/5 mL
5 Erythromycin suspension 300 mg	250 mg/5 mL
6 Digoxin suspension 125 microg	0.05 mg/mL
7 Phenytoin suspension 300 mg	125 mg/mL
8 Famotidine 60 mg	40 mg/5 mL

9 A child is ordered 25 mg of ibuprofen. The stock mixture on hand contains 100 mg in 5 mL. What volume of medication needs to be given to the child?

10 Hannah has been ordered 214 mg of amoxycillin. The mixture available contains 125 mg in 5 mL. What volume of medication needs to be given to the child?

11 Finlay is ordered 0.25 g of paracetamol. The stock strength on hand is 240 mg/5 mL. Calculate the amount required.

12 Eloise is to be given cephazolin 220 mg by injection. Stock vials contain 1 g in 10 mL after reconstitution. Calculate the volume to be given.

13 Michael is to receive 12 mg morphine. The stock ampoule contains 15 mg in 1 mL. What volume should be drawn up for the injection?

14 The stock strength of a drug is 500 mg in 2.5 mL. The prescriber has ordered 180 mg to be given as a stat dose. What volume would you give?

15 Your client is ordered ventolin syrup 6 mg every six hours. The syrup on hand is 2 mg/5 mL. What volume will you administer?

16 A client has been ordered 0.5 g of paracetamol PR. Stock available is 250 mg per suppository. How many suppositories should the client receive?

17 John is ordered 0.25 mg of clonazepam. 250 microg tablets are available. How many tablets will you give?

18 Mrs Gilmour is ordered a dose of 20 mg of frusemide. The stock available is 40 mg tablets. How many tablets will Mrs Gilmour receive?

19 Nick has a fever and is ordered 680 mg of paracetamol mixture. The strength in stock is 240 mg in 5 mL. What volume will you administer?

20 Thomas has been ordered 430 mg of amoxycillin suspension. The strength in stock is 500 mg in 5 mL. What volume would you administer?

21 A client is prescribed an injection of morphine 9 mg. The stock ampoule contains 15 mg in 1 mL. What volume should be drawn up for the injection?

22 Leo Branch is ordered 120 mg frusemide mane and 60 mg midday. Tablets are available in strengths of 20 mg, 40 mg and 500 mg. Which tablets would you use to make up these doses and how many would you administer?

23 Your brain-injured client is receiving 300 mg dilantin daily via an enteral feeding tube. Dilantin syrup is available as 30 mg/5 mL. How many mL will you administer?

24 You have 100 mg tablets of amiodarone available. Your client has been commenced on this antiarrhythmic agent 250 mg TDS.
   (a) How many tablets will the client receive in one dose?
   (b) How many tablets will the client receive per day?

25 An elderly client has been prescribed 12.5 mg felodipine for her hypertension. You have 10 mg tablets available. How many tablets will you administer?

26 Your client with pneumonia has been prescribed 550 mg of azithromycin daily. It is available to you as suspension 200 mg/5 mL. How many mL will you administer?

27 Your client has been ordered phytomenadione 12 mg as a pre-operative measure to treat a raised INR. To make up this dose you have available 2 mg/0.2 mL. How many mL will you administer?

28 Your client with severe, uncontrolled type 2 diabetes has had her metformin dose increased to 750 mg mane and lunch, and then 500 mg nocte. The available stock is 250 mg tablets. How many tablets will you administer for each dose?

29 Your client is in the acute phase of alcohol withdrawal. The doctor has prescribed oxazepam 15 mg QID. The available stock is 30 mg tablets. How many tablets will you administer for each dose?

30 A client with severe trigeminal neuralgia has been ordered daily carbamazepine 300 mg. The available stock is 200 mg. How many tablets will you administer?

31 Andrew is to be given flucloxacillin 275 mg by injection. Stock vials contain 1 g in 10 mL after dilution. Calculate the required volume to be administered.

32 Your client with unstable angina has been ordered isosorbide mononitrate XR 120 mg daily. Available tablets are 30 mg XR. How many tablets will you administer?

33 Fiona is receiving enteral feeds and has developed an acute duodenal ulcer. She has been commenced on esomeprazole IV. She weighs 18 kg. The dose rate is 2 mg/kg/day in divided doses 6 hourly. The stock strength is 25 mg/mL. How many mL will you administer in each dose?

34 A doctor has ordered a dopamine infusion to be run at 20 mg per hour. Dopamine is available in 400 mg ampoules and the protocol says to use a 500 mL bag of 5% glucose to make the solution. Calculate the rate of infusion.

35 A continuous infusion of heparin is running at 25 mL/h. The solution contains 40 000 units of heparin in 1 litre of solution. Calculate the dose of heparin that the client is receiving.

36 A solution of aminophylline is running at 80 mL/h. The solution contains 1 g diluted in 1 L of 5% glucose. Calculate the hourly amount being delivered to the client in mg.

37 A client has been ordered 10 mg/h of morphine. The solution has been prepared as 125 mg of morphine in 250 mL normal saline. Calculate the rate that needs to be given per hour to deliver the dose ordered.

38 A client is ordered isoproterenol to be infused at 4 microg/min. The available solution is 1 mg isoproterenol 250 mL 5% glucose. Calculate the flow rate needed to deliver the ordered dose.

39 A client (80 kg) is ordered a milrinone infusion at a rate of 0.5 microg/kg/min. The infusion is prepared with 10 mg milrinone in 50 mL normal saline. Calculate the rate in mL/h.

40 A client (90 kg) is ordered a glyceryl trinitrate (GTN) infusion at a rate of 5 microg/min. The infusion is prepared with 50 mg GTN in 500 mL 5% glucose. Calculate the rate in mL/h.

41 Ryan is a 26-month-old child who is to be commenced on digoxin for treatment of arrhythmia. He weighs 12 kg. His medication chart asks for one-half of the loading dose to be given stat, followed by one-quarter of the loading dose to be given 6 hours after, and the final dose to be given 12 hours after the initial dose. The total loading dose is 30 microg/kg. Digoxin mixture is available as 50 microg/mL.

    (a) Work out the total amount of digoxin to be given (in micrograms).

    (b) Calculate the initial loading dose in micrograms and by volume.

    (c) Calculate the volume of solution to be given at the 6- and 12-hour point.

42 Lynette Loughhead is a 24 kg child who is ordered benztropine. This preparation is to be given at a dose of 0.02 mg/kg/dose. What is the dose you would expect Lynette to be ordered?

43 Using the following formula, calculate the body surface area of Christopher Wines (height = 1.79 m, weight = 78 kg). Round the answer to one decimal point.

$$BSA(m^2) = \sqrt{\frac{ht(cm) \times wt(kg)}{3600}}$$

44 Calculate the creatinine clearance (CrCl) of Mr Pio Antonia, aged 65 years, using the formula from Chapter 1:

$$CrCl \ (mL/min) = \frac{(140 - age) \times weight \ (kg)}{0.814 \times serum \ creatinine \ (micromol/L)}$$

His serum creatinine is 455 micromol/L and his weight is 72 kg.

45 Write the following as mixed fractions:

a $\dfrac{52}{6}$

b $\dfrac{102}{4}$

46 Write the following ratios in fraction format:

a 4:1000

b 10:500

47 Convert the following decimal numbers to percentages:

a 0.78

b 0.92

48 Convert the following fractions to percentages:

a $\dfrac{6}{8}$

b $\dfrac{1}{5}$

49 Convert the following percentages to fractions:

a 16%

b 28%

50 An infusion has 400 mg of drug in 250 mL of diluent. What is the concentration in microg/mL?

51 An actrapid infusion has 50 units in 100 mL normal saline. What is the concentration in units/mL?

52 A client is ordered a 1000 mL Hartmann's flask over 6 hours. What is the rate in:

a drops per minute (assuming a macrodrip giving set)?

b mL/h?

53 A client is ordered 500 mL normal saline over 4 hours. What is the rate in:

a drops per minute (assuming a macrodrip giving set)?

b mL/h?

54 Amalie is ordered 15 mL of a medicine over 6 minutes. What is the rate in mL/h?

55 Aniela is ordered 20 mL of a medicine over 15 minutes. What is the rate in mL/h?

56 A 1-litre flask has been running at an 8-hourly rate for 2 hours via gravity feed. What is the rate in mL/h if you change to an infusion pump?

57 A 500 mL IV has been running for 2 hours at 42 drops per minute using a standard giving set. What is the rate in mL/h if you change to an infusion pump?

58 How long until these infusions finish:

a 1 litre over 12 hours started 4 hours ago?

b 500 mL over 1 hour started 45 minutes ago?

59 Calculate the amount of diluent required to make these medicines up to 10 mL:

a Antibiotic with powder volume 1.2 mL.

b Medicine with powder volume 0.7 mL.

60 Calculate the body surface area (BSA) for the following children using this formula from Chapter 7: (round answer to one decimal point)

$$\text{BSA(m}^2) = \sqrt{\frac{\text{ht(cm)} \times \text{wt(kg)}}{3600}}$$

a Elke weighs 52 kg and is 155 cm tall.

b Oliver weighs 43 kg and is 140 cm tall.

61 Calculate the rate (mL/h) to set for the following clients (weight = 70 kg):

a Dopamine at 8 microg/kg/min (infusion has 400 mg dopamine in 500 mL normal saline).

b Noradrenaline at 5 microg/min (infusion has 3 mg noradrenaline in 50 mL of 5% glucose).

Oncology

62 Calculate the body surface area (BSA) using the equations given in Chapter 10 for Ms Kerry Raynor, aged 55, who weighs 82 kg and is 170 cm tall. She is prescribed paclitaxel at 80 mg/m². Insert your answers in the following table.

	Body surface area (BSA) in m²	Required dose of paclitaxel in mg
Mosteller formula		
Du Bois formula		
Gehan and George formula		
Haycock formula		

Midwifery

63 Oxytocin is ordered as an infusion to contain 10 units of oxytocin in 1000 mL of normal saline. Oxytocin is available as 5 units/mL.

a What volume of oxytocin do you need to make up this infusion?

b What will you set the volume to be infused?

64 You need to administer naloxone 0.6 mg intravenously during an emergency. Naloxone ampoules contain 0.4 mg in 2 mL. What volume should be drawn up for injection?

65 A postpartum woman has been ordered 750 mg of an antibiotic for an infection. The medicine comes in a vial containing 1 g which needs to be made up to 10 mL with sterile water for injection. How much do you administer?

Medication chart questions

Using the included medication chart boxes, practise filling in the boxes based on the scenarios given.

Telephone orders

1   It is 6.15 p.m. on 21 October. A client in a private hospital has complained of nausea and vomiting following an anaesthetic. You phone her doctor, Dr Franke, who gives you a phone order for metoclopramide 10 mg IM once only. You ask another nurse to listen to the phone order also, and then fill out the medication chart.

Telephone orders (to be signed within 24 hours of order)													Record of administration			
Date time	Medicine (print generic name)	Route	Dose	Frequency	Check initials		Prescriber name	Pres. sign	Date	Time / given by	Time / given by	Time / given by	Time / given by
					N1	N2							

2   You are working in a small rural hospital on 15 June when the local GP, Dr Hecker, rings to order an antibiotic based on some pathology results that have arrived. He tells you that he will be able to come and see the client later that evening, and will write up the order then. It is currently 9.45 a.m. The doctor orders cephalexin 500 mg orally TDS. You ask another nurse to listen to the phone order also, and then complete the medication chart.

Telephone orders (to be signed within 24 hours of order)													Record of administration			
Date time	Medicine (print generic name)	Route	Dose	Frequency	Check initials		Prescriber name	Pres. sign	Date	Time / given by	Time / given by	Time / given by	Time / given by
					N1	N2							

Nurse-initiated medicines

3   Your client has asked for something for their headache. You notice that they have no medication ordered for pain relief. You also note that they have no known allergies. You decide to administer a nurse-initiated order for paracetamol 1 g, which is in accordance with your health service's policy. Fill out the medication chart.

Once only and nurse initiated medicines and pre-medications									
Date prescribed	Medicine (print generic name)	Route	**Dose**	Date/time of dose	Prescriber/Nurse Initiator (NI)		Given by	Time given	Pharmacy
					Signature	Print your name			

Nurse Initiated Medicine				Indication / instruction	Date	Time	Dose	Inits	Date	Time	Dose	Inits
Nurse Initiated Medicine			Strength									
Date	Route	Dose	Frequency									
/ /20												
RN Signature		RN Name (Print)										

4 Your client has been admitted for a routine test and they tell you they have a sore throat. They tell you that they have been taking throat lozenges at home, but they have not brought their medication with them. You decide to nurse-initiate a Cepacol lozenge and ask the doctor to review the client before they go home. Fill out the medication chart.

Once only and nurse initiated medicines and pre-medications								
Date prescribed	Medicine (print generic name)	Route	**Dose**	Date/time of dose	Prescriber/Nurse Initiator (NI) Signature Print your name		Given by	Time given	Pharmacy

ANSWERS

CHAPTER 1: BASIC MATHEMATICS

ACTIVITY 1.1
1   5 tablets
2   5 caplets
3   7 mL
4   3 tablets and 4 capsules; 7 medicines in total
5   7.5 mL

ACTIVITY 1.2
1   3 tablets
2   1 caplet
3   0.6 mL
4   3 capsules
5   194.5 mL

ACTIVITY 1.3
1   30 tablets
2   84 capsules
3   4 mL
4   25 mL

ACTIVITY 1.4
1   30 days
2   10 days
3   5 doses
4   10 hours
5   2 hours

ACTIVITY 1.5
1   45.67
2   30.08
3   26.23
4   9.04 mL/minute

ACTIVITY 1.6
1   $\dfrac{3}{24} = \dfrac{1}{8}$

2   $\dfrac{10}{24} = \dfrac{5}{12}$

3   $\dfrac{8}{24} = \dfrac{1}{3}$

ACTIVITY 1.7
1   $\dfrac{33}{4}$

2   $\dfrac{47}{16}$

3   $\dfrac{67}{2}$

4   $\dfrac{130}{8} = \dfrac{65}{4}$

5   $\dfrac{61}{7}$

ACTIVITY 1.8
1   $3\dfrac{3}{8}$

2   $7\dfrac{1}{5}$

3   $11\dfrac{1}{6}$

4   $7\dfrac{1}{3}$

5   $14\dfrac{1}{2}$

ACTIVITY 1.9
1   a $\dfrac{4}{10}$

   b $\dfrac{3}{6}$

   c $\dfrac{4}{8}$

   d $\dfrac{9}{12}$

   e $\dfrac{10}{16}$

   f $\dfrac{15}{27}$

2   a $\dfrac{6}{12}$

   b $\dfrac{3}{12}$

   c $\dfrac{12}{60}$

   d $\dfrac{63}{72}$

   e $\dfrac{32}{64}$

   f $\dfrac{12}{36}$

   g $\dfrac{10}{25}$

ACTIVITY 1.10
1   1
2   $\dfrac{1}{2}$
3   $\dfrac{1}{2}$
4   $\dfrac{1}{3}$
5   $\dfrac{13}{15}$

ACTIVITY 1.11
1   $\dfrac{7}{18}$
2   $\dfrac{1}{6}$
3   $\dfrac{9}{35}$
4   $\dfrac{2}{5}$
5   $\dfrac{13}{45}$

ACTIVITY 1.12
1   $\dfrac{1}{16}$
2   $\dfrac{3}{8}$

3   $\dfrac{4}{9}$
4   $\dfrac{21}{32}$
5   $\dfrac{49}{72}$

ACTIVITY 1.13
1   $\dfrac{4}{21}$
2   $\dfrac{10}{27}$
3   $3\dfrac{3}{5}$
4   $2\dfrac{1}{4}$
5   $4\dfrac{1}{6}$

ACTIVITY 1.14
1   $1\dfrac{2}{3}$
2   $1\dfrac{3}{5}$
3   1
4   $\dfrac{2}{7}$

5   $\dfrac{3}{5}$

ACTIVITY 1.15
1   $\dfrac{1}{12}$
2   $\dfrac{1}{40}$
3   $\dfrac{5}{12}$
4   $\dfrac{4}{15}$
5   $\dfrac{7}{16}$

ACTIVITY 1.16
1   $\dfrac{9}{40}$
2   $\dfrac{1}{3}$
3   $\dfrac{1}{9}$
4   $\dfrac{7}{16}$
5   $\dfrac{39}{112}$

ACTIVITY 1.17
1   115.252
2   169.3
3   4.849
4   117.0
5   152.95

ACTIVITY 1.18
1   9.1
2   6.29
3   5.9
4   2.87
5   7.9

ACTIVITY 1.19
1   0.35
2   0.006
3   0.045
4   7490
5   30.8

ACTIVITY 1.20
1   0.02
2   0.21
3   0.28
4   0.04
5   0.04

ACTIVITY 1.21
1   58
2   58

3   26
4   28
5   3

ACTIVITY 1.22
1   249.9
2   108.5
3   0.7
4   0.1
5   10.1

ACTIVITY 1.23
1   $10\dfrac{137}{1000}$
2   $\dfrac{933}{1000}$
3   $\dfrac{6}{25}$
4   $2\dfrac{3}{20}$
5   $\dfrac{3}{5}$

ACTIVITY 1.24
1   4.6
2   0.9
3   5.9
4   2.5
5   6.6

ACTIVITY 1.25

1 a 1:20
   b 5:20
   c 10:100
   d 25:100
   e 1:2

2 a $\dfrac{1}{2}$

   b $\dfrac{1}{2}$

   c $\dfrac{1}{20}$

   d $\dfrac{1}{10000}$

   e $\dfrac{4}{5}$

3 a 1:4
   b 2:3
   c 7:8
   d 3:4
   e 1:2

ACTIVITY 1.26

1 a 17%
   b 10%
   c 50%
   d 25%
   e 90%

2 a 0.16
   b 0.22
   c 0.55
   d 0.0005
   e 0.98

ACTIVITY 1.27

1 a 20%
   b 50%
   c 75%
   d 28%
   e 80%

2 a $\dfrac{9}{50}$

   b $\dfrac{7}{25}$

   c $\dfrac{57}{100}$

   d $\dfrac{47}{50}$

   e $\dfrac{1}{50}$

CHAPTER 2:
UNITS OF MEASUREMENT

ACTIVITY 2.1

1 a 0.014 g   e 400 g
   b 0.25 mg   f 3.2 L
   c 1500 mL   g 0.5 g
   d 1500 microg   h 0.125 mg

2 a 1000 mg, which is 2 tablets
   b 500 mg, which is 2 capsules
   c 125 microg, which is 2 tablets
   d 1200 mg, which is 3 tablets
   e 1250 mL

3 a 1200 mg
   b 700 mg
   c 50 microg
   d 2300 microg
   e 1070000 microg
   f 1400000 g
   g 0.006 mg is smaller
   h 0.06 mg is smaller
   i 6 microg is smaller
   j 0.0006 mg is smaller

ACTIVITY 2.2

1 a Administer 0.75 mL

b Administer 1.7 mL

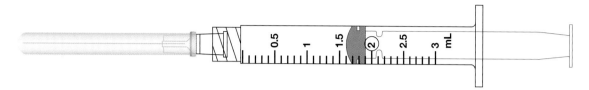

c Administer 2.2 mL

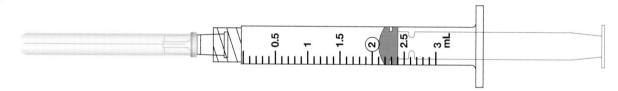

d Administer 1.3 mL

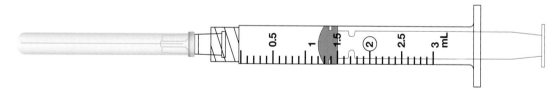

e Administer 0.33 mL

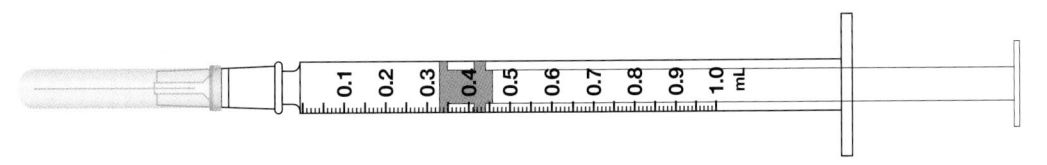

f Administer 65 units of insulin

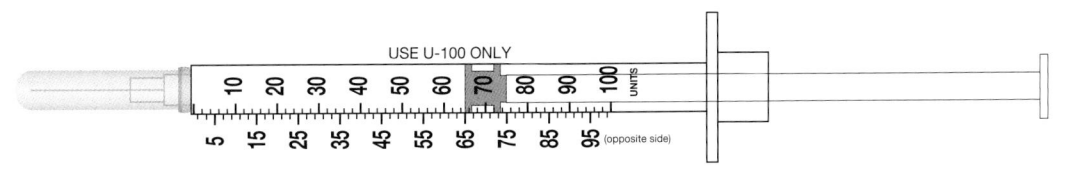

g Administer 27 units of insulin

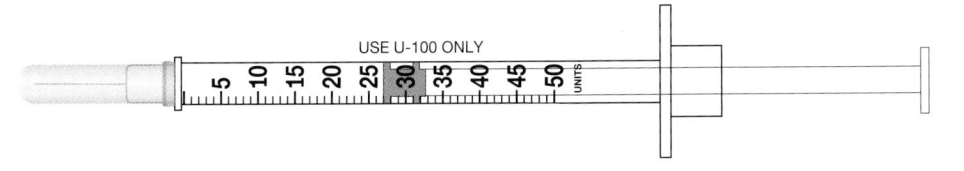

h Administer 75 units of insulin

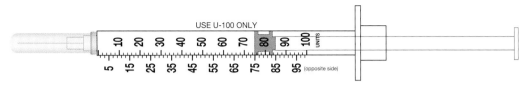

i Administer 4.4 mL

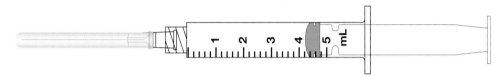

j Administer 16 mL

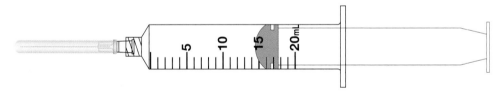

k 0.2 mL
l 1 mL
m 0.2 mL

2 a

b

3 a 7.5 mL
   b 2.5 mL
   c 4.0 mL
   d 7.4 mL

CHAPTER 3: MEDICATION CHARTS

ACTIVITY 3.1

1

Affix client identification label here
URN: *123456*
Family name: *Brown*   Not a valid
Given names: *Samantha*   prescription unless
Address: identifiers present
Date of birth: *13/1/19XX*   **Sex:** ☐ **M** ☒ **F**
First prescriber to print patient name and check label correct: *J Smith*

Affix client identification label here
URN: *654321*
Family name: *Brown*   Not a valid
Given names: *Samuel*   prescription unless
Address: identifiers present
Date of birth: *22/4/19XX*   **Sex:** ☒ **M** ☐ **F**
First prescriber to print patient name and check label correct: *J Smith*

- The clients could be given each other's medication without the nurse having the ability to check the identification of the correct client.
- Potential for anaphylaxis and death if one of the clients is allergic to the other's medications.
- Present medical conditions may not be treated by other person's medicine. In fact, this could lead to life-threatening ramifications. Mrs Brown would not be able to have surgery if she received antihypertensive or hypoglycaemic agents, or warfarin, which is used for atrial fibrillation.

2

Affix client identification label here
URN: *987654*
Family name: *Maher*
Given names: *Christopher*
Address:
Date of birth: *20/5/19XX*   **Sex:** ☒ **M** ☐ **F**
First prescriber to print patient name and check label correct: ___*J Smith*___

Not a valid prescription unless identifiers present

Affix client identification label here
URN: *456789*
Family name: *Maher*
Given names: *Christine*
Address:
Date of birth: *6/3/19XX*   **Sex:** ☐ **M** ☒ **F**
First prescriber to print patient name and check label correct: ___*J Smith*___

Not a valid prescription unless identifiers present

Potential outcomes for Christine:
- Anaphylaxis because she is allergic to penicillin.

Potential outcomes for Christopher:
- He may have adverse reactions to the other medicines on Christine's medication chart.

The areas in the patient identification panel that would prevent these errors from being made are:
- URN
- address
- date of birth
- sex/gender.

Note: any allergies will be recorded in the allergy section of the medication chart.

ACTIVITY 3.2

1

Facility/service:	Medicine chart no. .... of ....

Additional charts
☐ Iv fluid ☐ Bgl/insulin ☐ Acute pain ☐ Other
☐ Palliative care ☐ Chemotherapy ☐ Iv heparin

Ward/unit: ....

Once only and nurse initiated medicines and pre-medications

Date prescribed	Medicine (print generic name)	Route	Dose	Date/time of dose	Prescriber/Nurse Initiator (NI) Signature	Print your name	Given by	Time given	Pharmacy
21/9	Refresh tears	eye drop	1	21.9/1430	NJ	N. JAMES	SS	1435	

2

Facility/service:	Medicine chart no. .... of ....

Additional charts
☐ Iv fluid ☐ Bgl/insulin ☐ Acute pain ☐ Other
☐ Palliative care ☐ Chemotherapy ☐ Iv heparin

Ward/unit: ....

Once only and nurse initiated medicines and pre-medications

Date prescribed	Medicine (print generic name)	Route	Dose	Date/time of dose	Prescriber/Nurse Initiator (NI) Signature	Print your name	Given by	Time given	Pharmacy
14/4	Normal saline	IV	5 mL	14.4/1745	CJohns	C Johns	NJ	1800	

ACTIVITY 3.3

1

Telephone orders (to be signed within 24 hours of order)													
Date time	Medicine (print generic name)	Route	Dose	Frequency	Check initials		Prescriber name	Pres. sign	Date	Record of administration			
					N1	N2				Time / given by	Time / given by	Time / given by	Time / given by
15/10 /1000h	fexofenadine	PO	180 mg	mane	NJ	HW	Rose		15/10	1010 NJ			

ACTIVITY 3.4

1

Regular medicines

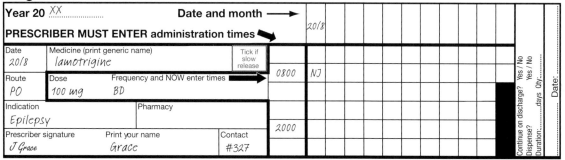

Year 20 XX

Date and month ———▶

PRESCRIBER MUST ENTER administration times ◀

20/8

Date 20/8	Medicine (print generic name) lamotrigine		Tick if slow release	0800	NJ			
Route PO	Dose 100 mg	Frequency and NOW enter times ▬▶ BD						
Indication Epilepsy		Pharmacy		2000				
Prescriber signature J Grace	Print your name Grace		Contact #327					

Continue on discharge? Yes / No
Dispense? Yes / No
Duration:........days Qty:.........
Date:

2   **Regular medicines**

Year 20 XX		Date and month ➞		20/8													Continue on discharge? Yes / No	Dispense? Yes / No	Date:
PRESCRIBER MUST ENTER administration times ➤																			
Date 20/8	Medicine (print generic name) bisoprolol		Tick if slow release																
Route PO	Dose 10 mg	Frequency and NOW enter times ➤ mane		0800	NJ												Duration:.......days Qty:.......		
Indication Hypertension		Pharmacy																	
Prescriber signature J Grace	Print your name Grace		Contact #327																

1

Date 17/8	Medicine (print generic name) morphine			Date 17/8													Continue on discharge? Yes / No	Dispense? Yes / No	
Route IM	Dose 5 mg	Hourly frequency 4/24 **PRN**	Max PRN dose/24 hrs 30 mg	Time 1100													......days Qty:.......		
Indication Pain		Pharmacy		Dose 5 mg															
				Route IM															
Prescriber signature J Grace	Print your name Grace		Contact #321	Sign TR													Duration:		

2

Date 17/8	Medicine (print generic name) metoclopramide			Date 17/8													Continue on discharge? Yes / No	Dispense? Yes / No	
Route IM	Dose 10 mg	Hourly frequency 6/24 **PRN**	Max PRN dose/24 hrs 40 mg	Time 1130													......days Qty:.......		
Indication Nausea		Pharmacy		Dose 10 mg															
				Route IM															
Prescriber signature J Grace	Print your name Grace		Contact #321	Sign TR													Duration:		

ACTIVITY 3.6

1

Date 15/8	Warfarin	(Marevan / Coumadin) select brand		INR Result	1.2	1.3	1.4	1.6	1.8						Continue on discharge? Yes / No Dispense? Yes / No Duration: .... days ...... Qty: .....
Route PO	Prescriber to enter individual doses	Target INR Range 2–3		**Dose**	2 mg	3 mg	3 mg	3 mg	3 mg	mg	mg	mg	mg	mg	
Indication Atrial fibrillation		Pharmacy		Prescriber	JG	JG	JG	JG	JG						
Prescriber signature J Grace	Print your name GRACE		Contact #321	1600 Initial 1	KR	NR	FM	AB	NR						
				Initial 2	VB	SM	CR	ZS	CR						

(column dates: 15/8 16/8 17/8 18/8 19/8)

2

Date 15/8	Warfarin	(Marevan / Coumadin) select brand		INR Result	1.2	1.3	1.4	1.6	1.8	2.1					Continue on discharge? Yes / No Dispense? Yes / No Duration: .... days ...... Qty: .....
Route PO	Prescriber to enter individual doses	Target INR Range 2–3		**Dose**	2 mg	3 mg	3 mg	3 mg	3 mg	2 mg	mg	mg	mg	mg	
Indication Atrial fibrillation		Pharmacy		Prescriber	JG	JG	JG	JG	JG	JG					
Prescriber signature J Grace	Print your name GRACE		Contact #321	1600 Initial 1	KR	NR	FM	AB	NR	NG					
				Initial 2	VB	SM	CR	ZS	CR	SR					

(column dates: 15/8 16/8 17/8 18/8 19/8 20/8)

ACTIVITY 3.7

1

Regular medicine

Year 20 XX	Date and month ⟶	21/8	22/8	23/8									
Variable dose medicine	Drug level												
Date	Medicine (print generic name)	Time level taken											
20/8	prednisolone	**Dose**	40 mg	35 mg	30 mg								
PO	Frequency: mane												
	Prescriber to enter dose times and individual dose	Prescriber	JG	JG	JG								
Indication: Asthma	Pharmacy	Time to be given: 0800	TR	TR									
Prescriber signature: J Grace	Print your name: Grace	Contact #321	Time given	0800	0800								

Continue on discharge? Yes / No — Dispense? Yes / No — Duration: _____ days — Qty: _____ — Date: _____

2

Regular medicine

Year 20 XX	Date and month ⟶	21/8	22/8	23/8									
Variable dose medicine	Drug level												
Date	Medicine (print generic name)	Time level taken											
20/8	prednisolone	**Dose**	40 mg	35 mg	30 mg								
PO	Frequency: mane												
	Prescriber to enter dose times and individual dose	Prescriber	JG	JG	JG								
Indication: Asthma	Pharmacy	Time to be given: 0800	TR	TR	TR								
Prescriber signature: J Grace	Print your name: Grace	Contact #321	Time given	0800	0800	0810							

Continue on discharge? Yes / No — Dispense? Yes / No — Duration: _____ days — Qty: _____ — Date: _____

CHAPTER 4: USING QUALITY AND RISK MANAGEMENT PRINCIPLES IN DOSAGE CALCULATIONS

ACTIVITY 4.1
1   1 tablet
2   8.3 mL
3   0.6 mL

CHAPTER 5: GENERAL DOSAGE CALCULATIONS

ACTIVITY 5.1
1   340–595 mg
2   325 mg
3   2790 mg

ACTIVITY 5.2
1    $\frac{1}{2}$ tablet
2   2 tablets
3    $\frac{1}{2}$ tablet

ACTIVITY 5.3
1   0.5 mg/g or 50 mg in total
2   50 g of dextrose
3   0.067 mg/mL

ACTIVITY 5.4
1   1.2 mL amoxycillin
2   6 mL gentamicin
3   6.5 mL amiodarone

CHAPTER 6: INFUSION CALCULATIONS

ACTIVITY 6.1
1   27.8 or 28 drops per minute
2   27.8 or 28 drops per minute
3   25 drops per minute

ACTIVITY 6.2
1   a   500 mL
     b   83 mL/h
2   a   100 mL
     b   50 mL/h
3   a   1000 mL
     b   83 mL/h

ACTIVITY 6.3
1   a   20 mL
     b   120 mL/h
2   a   10 mL
     b   20 mL/h
3   a   100 mL
     b   300 mL/h

ACTIVITY 6.4
1   a   41.67 or 42 mL/h
     b   790 mL
2   a   125 mL/h
     b   625 mL
3   a   28 drops per minute
     b   917 mL

ACTIVITY 6.5
1   500 mL to be infused over the next 2 hours
2   400 mL to be infused over the next 4 hours
3   850 mL to be infused over the next 8.5 hours

ACTIVITY 6.6
1   875 mL to be infused over the next 4 hours at 73 drops per minute
2   a   450 mL
     b   The new rate is 50 mL/h
     c   The infusion should end at 1730 hrs (9 hours later)
3   42 drops per minute

ACTIVITY 6.7
1   a   100 mL
     b   60 mL/h
2   a   2 mL/h
     b   48 mL fentanyl/24 h (i.e. 480 mcg of fentanyl/day)

CHAPTER 7: PAEDIATRIC CALCULATIONS

ACTIVITY 7.1
1   a   0.9 mg
     b   0.45 mL
2   a   60 mg
     b   0.6 mL
3   a   5.5 mg
     b   1.1 mL

ACTIVITY 7.2
1   0.82 m^2
2   0.29 m^2
3   0.57 m^2

ACTIVITY 7.3

1   a   8.6 mL of diluent
        gives 200 mg/mL
    b   7.5 mL to give 1.5 g
        IV
2   a   9.8 mL of diluent
        gives 25 mg/mL
    b   6 mL to give 150 g IV
3   a   8.8 mL of diluent
        gives 100 mg/mL
    b   7.5 mL to give 750 mg
        IV

ACTIVITY 7.4

1   0.85 m²
2   2.5 mL salbutamol
    6.9 mL paracetamol
    5.5 mL flucloxacillin

CHAPTER 8: MIDWIFERY CALCULATIONS

ACTIVITY 8.1

1   a   0.7 mL of
        concentrated fentanyl
        2 mL metoclopramide
    b   4 mL of oxytocin goes
        into the Hartmanns
        solution; the infusion
        rate is 251 mL/h
        0.5 mL ergometrine

    c   0.1 mL
        phytomenadione IM

CHAPTER 9: CRITICAL CARE AND HIGH DEPENDENCY DOSAGE CALCULATIONS

ACTIVITY 9.1

1   0.9 mL/h
2   9 mL/h
3   90 mL/h

ACTIVITY 9.2

1   14.6 mL/h
2   24.9 mL/h
3   3.4 mL/h

ACTIVITY 9.3

1   a   4 mL bolus
    b   48 mL/h
2   a   5 mL bolus
    b   30 mL/h
3   a   10 mL bolus
    b   999 mL/h

ACTIVITY 9.4

1   a   0.84 microg/min
    b   1209.5 microg in total
        for 24 h
    c   20 microg/mL
    d   2.5 mL/h

e

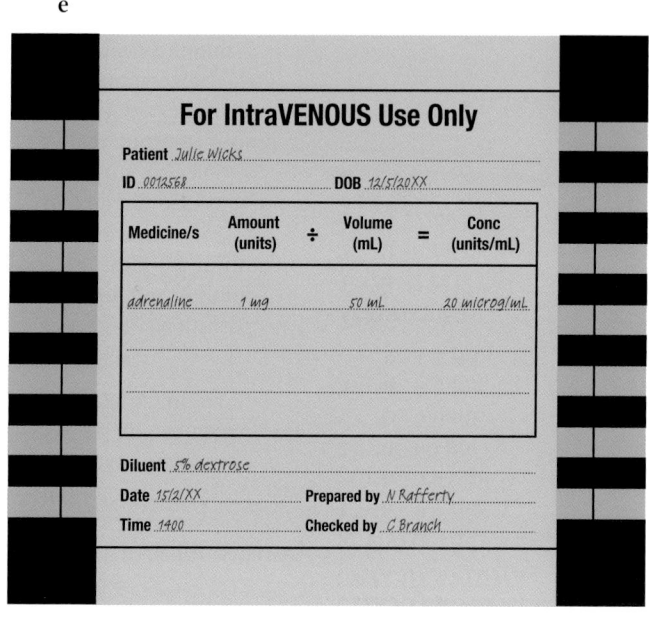

2   a   164 mcg/min
    b   236.16 mg/day
    c   1.64 mL/h

d

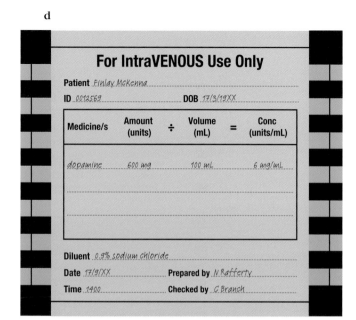

For IntraVENOUS Use Only

Patient *Finlay McKenna*

ID *0012569*   DOB *17/3/19XX*

Medicine/s	Amount (units)	÷	Volume (mL)	=	Conc (units/mL)
dopamine	*600 mg*		*100 mL*		*6 mg/mL*

Diluent *0.9% sodium chloride*

Date *17/9/XX*   Prepared by *N Rafferty*

Time *1400*   Checked by *C Branch*

CHAPTER 10: OTHER SPECIALIST AREAS: AGED CARE, MENTAL HEALTH AND ONCOLOGY

ACTIVITY 10.1

1   $\frac{1}{2}$ tablet atenolol

42 mL phenytoin

4 mL frusemide

$\frac{1}{2}$ tablet digoxin

$\frac{1}{2}$ tablet enalapril

2 tablets diclofenac (check with prescriber as enteric-coated tablets cannot be crushed)

ACTIVITY 10.2

1   2 tablets of diazepam (PRN)

0.5 mL haloperidol (PRN)

$\frac{1}{2}$ tablet of chlorpromazine

2 tablets of lithium

ACTIVITY 10.3

1   **MOSTELLAR FORMULA**

1.75 m^2

DU BOIS FORMULA

1.75 m^2

GEHAN AND GEORGE FORMULA

1.76 m^2

HAYCOCK FORMULA

1.75 m^2

2   105 mg doxorubicin

3   52.5 mL doxorubicin

4   410 mL/h

PRACTICE QUESTIONS:

BASIC MATHEMATICS

BASIC ARITHMETIC

1 19
2 74
3 492
4 1113
5 423
6 435
7 87
8 2238
9 4824
10 65
11 1328
12 648
13 12792
14 218340
15 712008
16 11
17 14
18 75
19 63
20 93

FRACTIONS AND DECIMALS

21 $\dfrac{1}{3}$

22 $\dfrac{1}{40}$

23 $\dfrac{1}{3}$

24 $12\dfrac{1}{2}$

25 $4\dfrac{11}{15}$

26 $5\dfrac{2}{5}$

27 $2\dfrac{3}{8}$

28 $3\dfrac{5}{6}$

29 $6\dfrac{1}{2}$

30 $1\dfrac{5}{18}$

31 $\dfrac{1}{69}$

32 $\dfrac{85}{207}$

33 $\dfrac{7}{32}$

34 $\dfrac{2}{27}$

35 $\dfrac{7}{55}$

36 $\dfrac{5}{8}$

37 $\dfrac{11}{18}$

38 $\dfrac{15}{22}$

39 $1\dfrac{1}{8}$

40 $\dfrac{26}{33}$

41 0.86
42 0.88
43 0.26
44 0.61
45 0.17
46 2.501
47 0.098
48 0.096
49 8.057
50 5.281
51 82.82
52 3.778
53 8.31
54 60.32

55 26.74
56 6198.3
57 464.62
58 568.42
59 283.22
60 768.69
61 1.70
62 9.03
63 0.14
64 1.90
65 25.25

CONVERSION

66 a 0.475 g
    b 3.75 L
    c 0.245 mg
    d 0.75 g
    e 35 000 mg
    f 750 000 microg

GENERAL QUESTIONS

1 3 mL
2 8.3 mL
3 2.5 mL
4 3.1 mL
5 6 mL
6 2.5 mL
7 2.4 mL
8 7.5 mL
9 1.25 mL

10 8.56 mL − rounded
    up to 8.6 mL
11 5.2 mL
12 2.2 mL
13 0.8 mL
14 0.9 mL
15 15 mL
16 2 suppositories
17 1 tablet
18 0.5 tablets
19 14.2 mL
20 4.3 mL
21 0.6 mL
22 Mane: 3×40 mg;
    midday: 1×40 mg
    and 1×20 mg
23 50 mL
24 a 2.5 tablets
    b 7.5 tablets
25 $1\frac{1}{4}$ tablets
26 13.75 mL
27 1.2 mL
28 3 tablets mane, 3 tablets lunch
    and 2 tablets nocte
29 0.5 tablets
30 1.5 tablets
31 2.75 mL
32 4 tablets

33 0.36 mL/dose
34 25 mL/h
35 1000 units/h
36 80 mg
37 20 mL/h
38 60 mL/h
39 12 mL/h
40 3 mL/h
41 a 360 microg digoxin
    b The initial loading
       dose of digoxin is
       180 microg and the volume is
       3.6 mL
    c 1.8 mL digoxin
42 0.48 mg
43 2.0 m²
44 14.58 mL/min
45 a $8\frac{2}{3}$
    b $25\frac{1}{2}$
46 a $\frac{1}{250}$
    b $\frac{1}{50}$
47 a 78%
    b 92%

48 a 75%
    b 20%
49 a $\frac{4}{25}$
    b $\frac{7}{25}$
50 1600 microg/mL
51 0.5 units/mL
52 a 55.5 or 56 drops per minute
    b 166.67 mL per hour or
       167 mL per hour (rounded up)
53 a 41.66 or 42 drops per minute
    b 125 mL/h
54 150 mL/h
55 80 mL/h
56 125 mL/h
57 125 mL/h
58 a 8 h
    b 15 mins remaining
59 a 8.8 mL
    b 9.3 mL
60 a 1.5 m²
    b 1.3 m²
61 a 42 mL/h
    b 5 mL/h

ONCOLOGY

62

	Body surface area (BSA) in m^2	Required dose of paclitaxel in mg
Mosteller formula	1.967 m^2	157.4 mg
Du Bois formula	1.936 m^2	154.9 mg
Gehan and George formula	1.987 m^2	159.0 mg
Haycock formula	1.988 m^2	159.0 mg

MIDWIFERY

63 **a** 2 mL
     b 1000 mL

64 3 mL

65 7.5 mL

MEDICATION CHART QUESTIONS

TELEPHONE ORDERS

1

Telephone orders (to be signed within 24 hours of order)													
Date time	Medicine (print generic name)	Route	Dose	Frequency	Check initials N1	Check initials N2	Prescriber name	Pres. sign	Date	Time / given by	Time / given by	Time / given by	Time / given by
21/10 1815	METOCLOPRAMIDE	IM	10 mg	STAT	KR	VB	DISH			1820 KR			

2

					Check initials					Record of administration			
Date time	Medicine (print generic name)	Route	Dose	Frequency	N1	N2	Prescriber name	Pres. sign	Date	Time / given by	Time / given by	Time / given by	Time / given by

Telephone orders (to be signed within 24 hours of order)

Date time	Medicine (print generic name)	Route	Dose	Frequency	N1	N2	Prescriber name	Pres. sign	Date	Time / given by	Time / given by	Time / given by	Time / given by
15/6 0945	CEPHALEXIN	PO	500 mg	TDS	KR	VB	SMITH			0950 KR			

NURSE-INITIATED MEDICINES

3

Once only and nurse initiated medicines and pre-medications

Date prescribed	Medicine (print generic name)	Route	Dose	Date/time of dose	Prescriber/Nurse Initiator (NI) Signature	Print your name	Given by	Time given	Pharmacy
24/8/XX	PARACETAMOL	PO	1 g	24/8/19 1800	*(signature)*	RAFFERTY	KR	1810	

Nurse Initiated Medicine		Indication / instruction	Date	Time	Dose	Inits	Date	Time	Dose	Inits
Nurse Initiated Medicine Paracetamol	Strength 500 mg	Headache	24/8	1810 h	1 g	KR				
Date 24/8/20XX	Route PO	Dose 1 g	Frequency 4–6 hrly							
RN Signature *(signature)*		RN Name (Print) K Rafferty								

4

Once only and nurse initiated medicines and pre-medications

Date prescribed	Medicine (print generic name)	Route	Dose	Date/time of dose	Prescriber/Nurse Initiator (NI) Signature	Print your name	Given by	Time given	Pharmacy
1/7/XX	CEPACOL LOZENGE	TOP	1	1/7/19 2100	*(signature)* J Branch	J BRANCH	JB	2110	

REFERENCES

Australian Bureau of Statistics (2023). *Population projections, Australia 2022 (base)–2071*. https://www.abs.gov.au/statistics/people/population/population-projections-australia

Australian Commission on Safety and Quality in Health Care (2013a). *Literature Review: Medication Safety in Australia*. ACSQHC, Sydney.

Australian Commission on Safety and Quality in Health Care (2013b). *National Recommendations for User-applied Labelling of Injectable Medicines, Fluids and Lines*. ACSQHC, Sydney.

Australian Commission on Safety and Quality in Health Care (2023). *Atlas 2021, 6.1 Polypharmacy, 75 years and over*. https://www.safetyandquality.gov.au/our-work/healthcare-variation/fourth-atlas-2021/medicines-use-older-people/61-polypharmacy-75-years-and-over

Australian Commission on Safety and Quality in Health Care (2024). *Action 4.10: Medication Review*. https://www.safetyandquality.gov.au/standards/nsqhs-standards/medication-safety-standard/continuity-medication-management/action-410

Australian Government Cancer Australia EdCaN (2024). Cancer learning topics. https://www.cancerlearning.gov.au/topics/edcan

Australian Government Department of Health and Aged Care (2022). *National Medicines Policy*. https://www.health.gov.au/resources/publications/national-medicines-policy

Australian Injectable Drugs Handbook, 9th edn (2023). The Society of Hospital Pharmacists of Australia, https://aidh.hcn.com.au

Australian Institute of Health and Welfare (AIHW) (2021). Cancer in Australia 2021, 1 December. https://www.aihw.gov.au/reports/cancer/cancer-in-australia-2021/summary

Australian Institute of Health and Welfare (AIHW) (2023a). Older Australians: Health – selected conditions, updated 18 June. https://www.aihw.gov.au/reports/older-people/older-australians/contents/health/health-disability-status

Australian Institute of Health and Welfare (AIHW) (2023b). Prevalence and impact of mental illness. https://www.aihw.gov.au/mental-health/overview/prevalence-and-impact-of-mental-illness

Australian Medicines Handbook. https://amhonline.amh.net.au/

Cancer Council Australia (2023). Clinical Guidelines: How is dosage of cancer therapy calculated for adults? https://wiki.cancer.org.au/australia/Clinical_question:How_is_dosage_of_cancer_therapy_calculated_for_adults%3F

Commonwealth of Australia (2022). *Guiding Principles for Medication Management in the Community*. https://www.health.gov.au/resources/collections/guiding-principles-for-medication-management-in-the-community-collection

Dementia Australia (2023). Drugs used to relieve behavioural & psychological symptoms of dementia. https://www.dementia.org.au/information/about-dementia/what-is-dementia how-is-dementia-treated/drugs-used-to-relieve-behavioural-psychological-symptoms-of-dementia

DuBois, D. & DuBois, E.F. (1916). A formula to estimate the approximate surface area if height and weight be known. *Archives of Internal Medicine*, 17(6-2), pp. 863–71.

eviQ Cancer Institute of NSW (n.d.a). Body surface area calculator. https://www.eviq.org.au/clinical-resources/eviq-calculators/3198-body-surface-area-calculator

eviQ Cancer Institute of NSW (n.d.b). Clinical procedure – administration of anti-cancer drugs – intramuscular and subcutaneous. https://www.eviq.org.au/clinical-resources/administration-of-anti-cancer-drugs/457-administration-of-anti-cancer-drugs-intramus#procedure

Flenady, V., Wojcieszek, A.M., Papatsonis, D.N.M., Stock, O.M., Murray, L., Jardine, L.A. & Carbonne, B. (2014). Calcium channel blockers for inhibiting preterm labour and birth. *Cochrane Database of Systematic Reviews*, Issue 6. Art. No.: CD002255. DOI: 10.1002/14651858.CD002255.pub2

Gehan, E.A. & George, S.L. (1970). Estimation of human body surface area from height and weight. *Cancer Chemotherapy Reports*, 54, pp. 225–35.

Greenfield, S., Whelan, B. & Cohn, E. (2006). Use of dimensional analysis to reduce medication errors. *Journal of Nursing Education*, 45(2), pp. 91–4.

Haycock, G.B., Schwartz, G.J. & Wisotsky, D.H. (1978). Geometric method for measuring body surface area: A height-weight formula validated in infants, children and adults. *The Journal of Pediatrics*, 93(1), pp. 62–6.

Jordan, S. (2010). *Pharmacology for Midwives. The evidence base for safe practice*, 2nd edn. Palgrave Macmillan, Basingstoke.

Kliegman, R.M., Stanton, B.M.D., St. Geme, J., Schor, N. & Behrman, R.E. (eds) (2011). *Nelson Textbook of Pediatrics*, 19th edn. Saunders, Elsevier, Philadelphia.

Likis, F.E., Andrews, J.C., Collins, M.R., Lewis, R.M., Seroogy, J.J., Starr, S.A., Walden, R.R. & McPheeters, M.L. (2014). Nitrous oxide for the management of labor pain: A systematic review. *Anesthesia & Analgesia*, 118(1), pp. 153–67.

Mosteller, R.D. (1987). Simplified calculation of body surface area. *The New England Journal of Medicine*, 317(17), p. 1098 (letter).

National Physical Laboratory (2010). *What are the Differences Between Mass, Weight, Force and Load?* http://www.npl.co.uk/reference/faqs/what-are-the-differences-between-mass,-weight,-force-and-load-(faq-mass-and-density)

Royal Australian and New Zealand College of Obstetricians and Gynaecologists (2016). Pain relief in labour and childbirth. https://www.ranzcog.edu.au/RANZCOG_SITE/media/RANZCOG-MEDIA/Women%27s%20Health/Patient%20information/Pain-relief-labour-childbirth-pamphlet.pdf?ext=.pdf

Stats NZ Tatauranga Aotearoa (2022). New Zealanders' mental wellbeing declines, 5 July. https://www.stats.govt.nz/news/new-zealanders-mental-wellbeing-declines

Stefani, M., Singer, R.F. & Roberts D.M. (2019). How to adjust drug doses in chronic kidney disease. *Australian Prescriber*, 42, pp. 163–7. https://australianprescriber.tg.org.au/articles/how-to-adjust-drug-doses-in-chronic-kidney-disease.html

Te Tahu Hauora Health Quality & Safety Commission (2023). *Reducing Harm: Medicines.* https://www.hqsc.govt.nz/our-work/system-safety/reducing-harm/medicines

World Health Organization (2023). Medication without harm. https://www.who.int/initiatives/medication-without-harm

World Health Organization (2024). Health topics: Mental health. https://www.who.int/health-topics/mental-health#tab=tab_2

INDEX